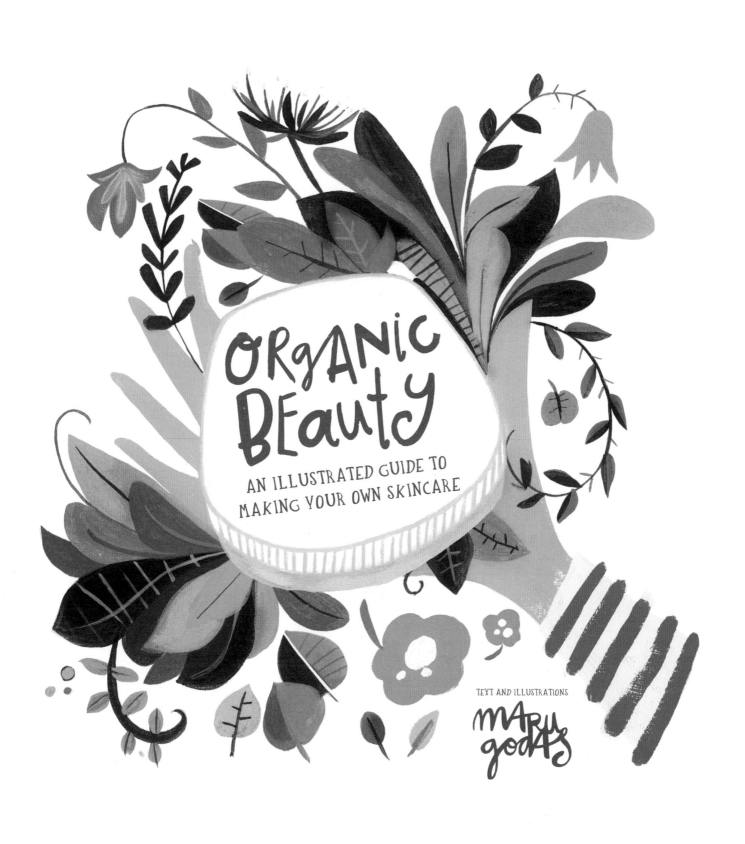

# ORGANIC BEAUTY

## AN ILLUSTRATED GUIDE TO MAKING YOUR OWN SKINCARE

TEXT AND ILLUSTRATIONS

MARU godAS

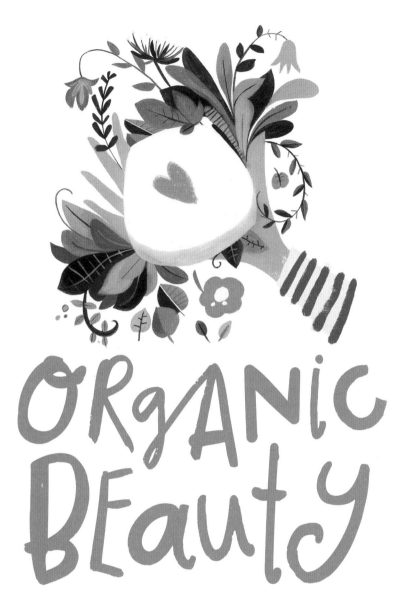

# ORGANIC BEAUTY

## AN ILLUSTRATED GUIDE TO MAKING YOUR OWN SKINCARE

TEXT AND ILLUSTRATIONS

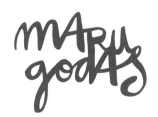

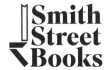
Smith
Street
Books

# CONTENTS

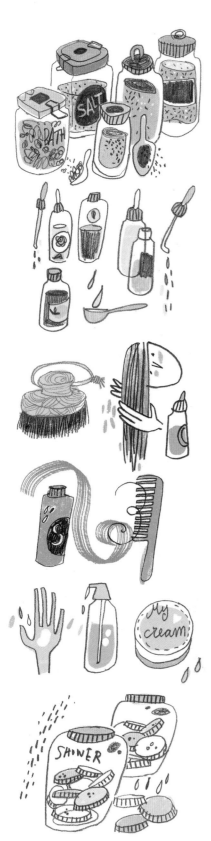

Drawn with love and passion 6
  Beauty comes from the inside out 8
  Loving our bodies 11
  Why natural cosmetics? 12
  What's in my cream? 13

The plants 14
  The illustrated herbarium 16
  Collection and preservation 24
  Plant preparations 26

Vegetable oils and fats 30
  Vegetable oils in cosmetics 32
  Vegetable butters and waxes 38

Essential oils 40
  Floral essential oils 42
  Citrus essential oils 44
  Herbaceous essential oils 46
  Tree essential oils 48
  Precautions and uses of essential oils 50
  Essential oils and emotions 52

Fruits, vegetables and fresh products 54
  From the garden to your skin:
    fruits and vegetables 56
  Cosmetics from your kitchen 58

Let's get to work! The recipes 60
  Before starting 62
  Guidance tables 63
  Utensils 64
  Raw materials 65

Face masks 66
  Fifteen minutes of love 68
  Dear clays 69

Exfoliants 70
  Facial scrubs 72
  Body scrubs 74

Baths 76
   Body baths 78
   Effervescent bath bombs 80
   Foot baths 81
   Shower discs 81

Oils and serums 82
   Facial cleansing with vegetable oils 84
   Facial oils 86
   Macerated oils 87
   Body oils 88

Balms and butters 90
   Step-by-step: balms 92
   Lip balms 93
   Balms with infused oils 95
   Solid moisturisers 96
   Body butters 97

Hydrosols and floral waters 98
   Infusions and waters 100
   Hydrosols and skin types 101

Creams and lotions 102
   Basic emulsion 104
   Creams 106

Hair care 108
   Step-by-step: henna dye 110
   A la carte shampoos 112

Deodorants and oral care 114
   Deodorants 116
   Oral care 117

Soaps 118
   Castile soap 120

Extras 122

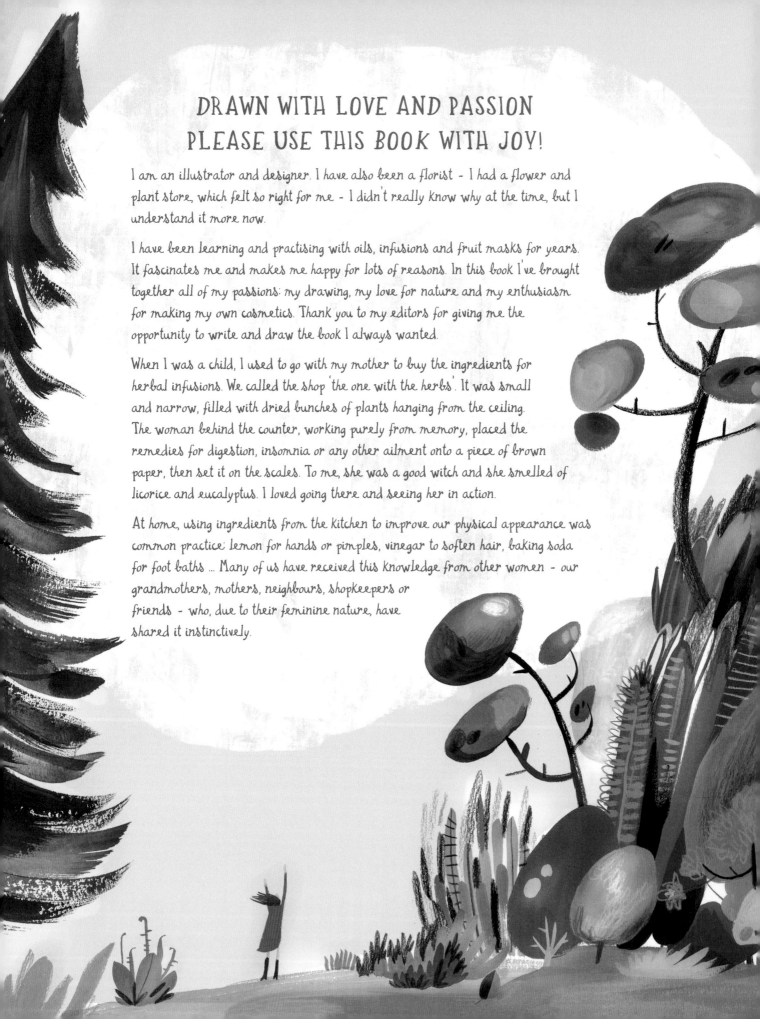

# DRAWN WITH LOVE AND PASSION
# PLEASE USE THIS BOOK WITH JOY!

I am an illustrator and designer. I have also been a florist - I had a flower and plant store, which felt so right for me - I didn't really know why at the time, but I understand it more now.

I have been learning and practising with oils, infusions and fruit masks for years. It fascinates me and makes me happy for lots of reasons. In this book I've brought together all of my passions: my drawing, my love for nature and my enthusiasm for making my own cosmetics. Thank you to my editors for giving me the opportunity to write and draw the book I always wanted.

When I was a child, I used to go with my mother to buy the ingredients for herbal infusions. We called the shop 'the one with the herbs'. It was small and narrow, filled with dried bunches of plants hanging from the ceiling. The woman behind the counter, working purely from memory, placed the remedies for digestion, insomnia or any other ailment onto a piece of brown paper, then set it on the scales. To me, she was a good witch and she smelled of licorice and eucalyptus. I loved going there and seeing her in action.

At home, using ingredients from the kitchen to improve our physical appearance was common practice: lemon for hands or pimples, vinegar to soften hair, baking soda for foot baths ... Many of us have received this knowledge from other women - our grandmothers, mothers, neighbours, shopkeepers or friends - who, due to their feminine nature, have shared it instinctively.

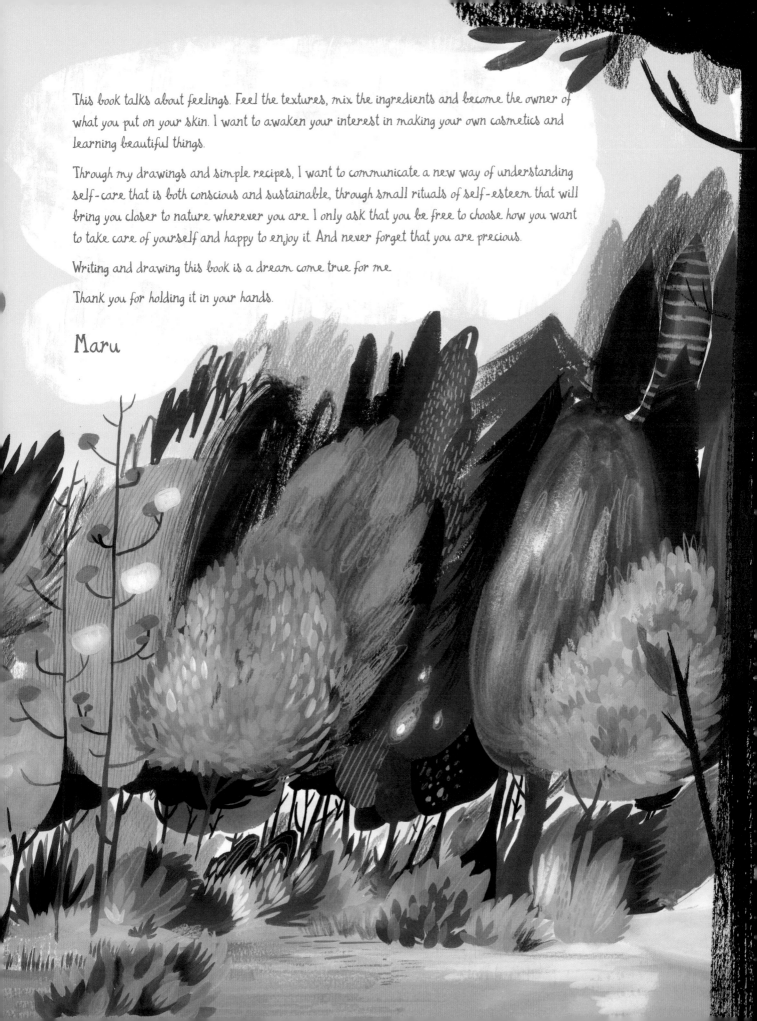

This book talks about feelings. Feel the textures, mix the ingredients and become the owner of what you put on your skin. I want to awaken your interest in making your own cosmetics and learning beautiful things.

Through my drawings and simple recipes, I want to communicate a new way of understanding self-care that is both conscious and sustainable, through small rituals of self-esteem that will bring you closer to nature wherever you are. I only ask that you be free to choose how you want to take care of yourself and happy to enjoy it. And never forget that you are precious.

Writing and drawing this book is a dream come true for me.

Thank you for holding it in your hands.

Maru

# BEAUTY COMES FROM THE INSIDE OUT

Beauty comes from the inside out. That's how nature works.

We all know that our face and eyes, the mirrors of our souls, reflect what is happening inside us. We look in the mirror and quickly reach for make-up or blush to help hide that tired and sad look, but we often don't reflect on what we are thinking or feeling.

Emotions such as anger or sadness are directly reflected on our face through wrinkles, bags or dark circles. Our skin 'feels' and expresses itself with the help of thousands of nerve endings, sometimes responding with diseases associated with stress such as psoriasis, eczema or dermatitis. But when our skin is caressed, hugged and kissed, it is radiant and we shine.

In addition to poor diet, a sedentary life and lack of sleep, negative emotions appear on our face, visible through our make-up. Given this, my proposal is that we start from the inside: review our emotional beauty, our diet and our sleep to help us feel beautiful.

A daily yoga or stretching routine, an energising shower, a walk in the park, a litre of water, a good book, a healthy meal in good company, laughing with friends … all of this beautifies us and is reflected on our face. It's like a serum of happiness.

Before explaining the recipes and beauty tricks, I want to first ask you to respect your own priorities rather than sacrifice your emotional care for things that, although important, are not fundamental.

Being well inside comes first.

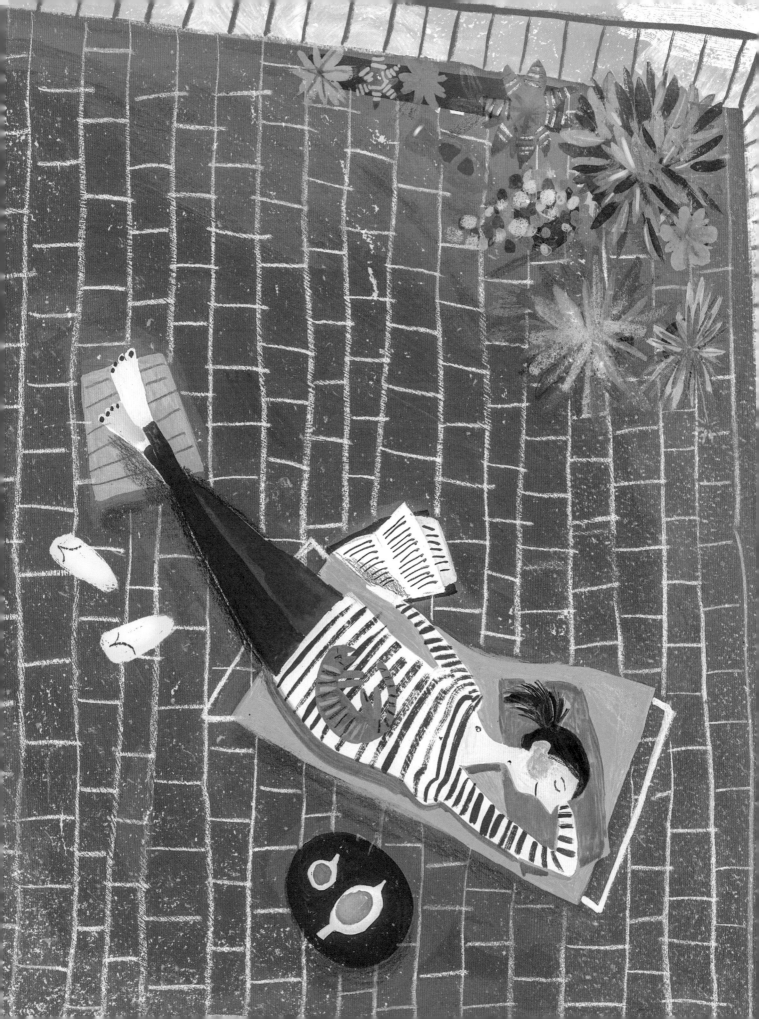

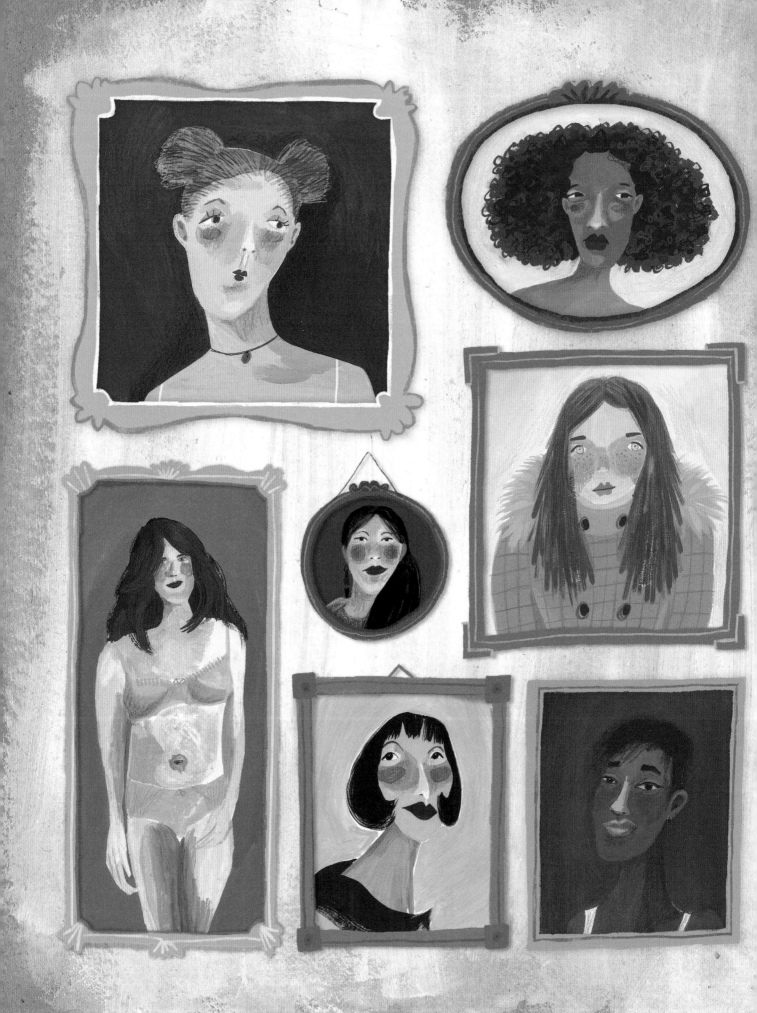

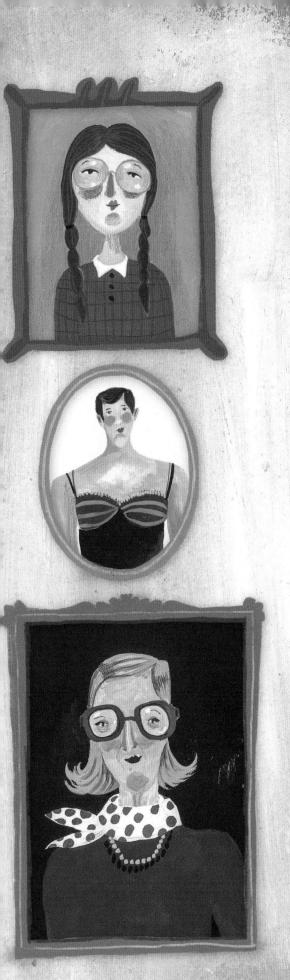

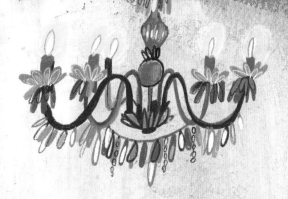

# LOVING OUR BODIES

We all want to feel beautiful.

That poetic concept has been and continues to be a burden for many of us. It seems that it is important for women to live under the pressure of ideals that are impossible to achieve and to deny our bodies.

Every day, we are bombarded by messages telling us we need to use beauty products. We know that there are companies whose only objectives are economic – they do not always respect ethical limits, nor do they take into account the side effects of their products on our health or our environment. I ask you to reflect on that.

Taking care of our appearance and our bodies should be an act of love for ourselves, claimed from the feminine identity, whether we are big, short, skinny, with or without breasts. Regardless of our age, skin colour, lifestyle or sexual orientation, we are all beautiful if we feel free and happy.

Luckily, it seems that we are winning the battle against stereotypes by empowering ourselves and claiming 'imperfect beauty', along with all the characteristics that we know make us unique.

My proposal is that you take care of yourself and pamper yourself, that you enjoy your little rituals, that you share them with the people you love and that you use clean products, free of unnecessary chemicals.

The first step towards loving our body is to take care of it by using what is closest to where we come from – nature.

# WHY NATURAL COSMETICS?

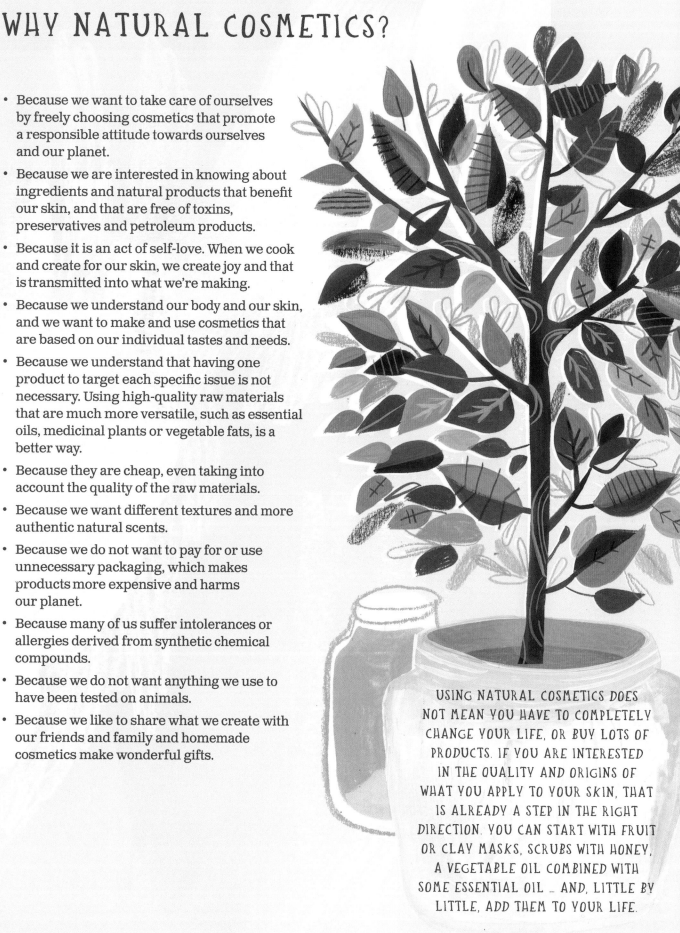

- Because we want to take care of ourselves by freely choosing cosmetics that promote a responsible attitude towards ourselves and our planet.

- Because we are interested in knowing about ingredients and natural products that benefit our skin, and that are free of toxins, preservatives and petroleum products.

- Because it is an act of self-love. When we cook and create for our skin, we create joy and that is transmitted into what we're making.

- Because we understand our body and our skin, and we want to make and use cosmetics that are based on our individual tastes and needs.

- Because we understand that having one product to target each specific issue is not necessary. Using high-quality raw materials that are much more versatile, such as essential oils, medicinal plants or vegetable fats, is a better way.

- Because they are cheap, even taking into account the quality of the raw materials.

- Because we want different textures and more authentic natural scents.

- Because we do not want to pay for or use unnecessary packaging, which makes products more expensive and harms our planet.

- Because many of us suffer intolerances or allergies derived from synthetic chemical compounds.

- Because we do not want anything we use to have been tested on animals.

- Because we like to share what we create with our friends and family and homemade cosmetics make wonderful gifts.

USING NATURAL COSMETICS DOES NOT MEAN YOU HAVE TO COMPLETELY CHANGE YOUR LIFE, OR BUY LOTS OF PRODUCTS. IF YOU ARE INTERESTED IN THE QUALITY AND ORIGINS OF WHAT YOU APPLY TO YOUR SKIN, THAT IS ALREADY A STEP IN THE RIGHT DIRECTION. YOU CAN START WITH FRUIT OR CLAY MASKS, SCRUBS WITH HONEY, A VEGETABLE OIL COMBINED WITH SOME ESSENTIAL OIL ... AND, LITTLE BY LITTLE, ADD THEM TO YOUR LIFE.

# WHAT'S IN MY CREAM?

I propose that you choose brands that respect the ingredients in their products and use sustainable manufacturing processes. Here are some guidelines to help identify them.

INCI (International Nomenclature of Cosmetic Ingredients) is the international naming convention by which the ingredients of products must be termed in their labelling. I've summarised the basic points so that you can review labels and check if a product or brand follows the legislation:

- Ingredients must be listed in order of concentration, from largest to smallest. Those listed first are the main ingredients in the product.

- Ingredients with a concentration of less than 1% may be listed in any order after the main ingredients. Some brands deliberately group these, so that the prized ingredients are not listed last, even though they are only present in small amounts.

- Ingredients from plants must be written using the plant's Latin (or scientific) name. Other compounds are named by their scientific name. Be careful: not all chemical compounds are toxic.

In addition to the INCI, there are other 'seals' for natural and ecological cosmetics, which guarantee the quality and origin of the products they appear on. These seals, or logos, are printed on the product's packaging. They include COSMOS, Natrue, Ecocert, Cosmebio, Demeter, IMO, Soil Association, and USDA Organic and Natural Products Association. They are all slightly different in terms of what they guarantee about the amount of raw materials of natural origin and the ecological impacts of the product.

Finally, the Leaping Bunny or 'jumping rabbit' logo (managed by the Coalition for Consumer Information on Cosmetics) certifies that no animal tests have been carried out at any stage in the manufacture of a product.

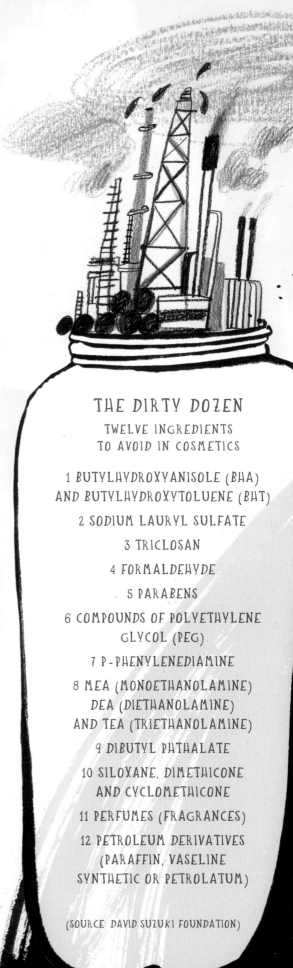

## THE DIRTY DOZEN
### TWELVE INGREDIENTS TO AVOID IN COSMETICS

1 BUTYLHYDROXYANISOLE (BHA) AND BUTYLHYDROXYTOLUENE (BHT)

2 SODIUM LAURYL SULFATE

3 TRICLOSAN

4 FORMALDEHYDE

5 PARABENS

6 COMPOUNDS OF POLYETHYLENE GLYCOL (PEG)

7 P-PHENYLENEDIAMINE

8 MEA (MONOETHANOLAMINE) DEA (DIETHANOLAMINE) AND TEA (TRIETHANOLAMINE)

9 DIBUTYL PHTHALATE

10 SILOXANE, DIMETHICONE AND CYCLOMETHICONE

11 PERFUMES (FRAGRANCES)

12 PETROLEUM DERIVATIVES (PARAFFIN, VASELINE SYNTHETIC OR PETROLATUM)

(SOURCE: DAVID SUZUKI FOUNDATION)

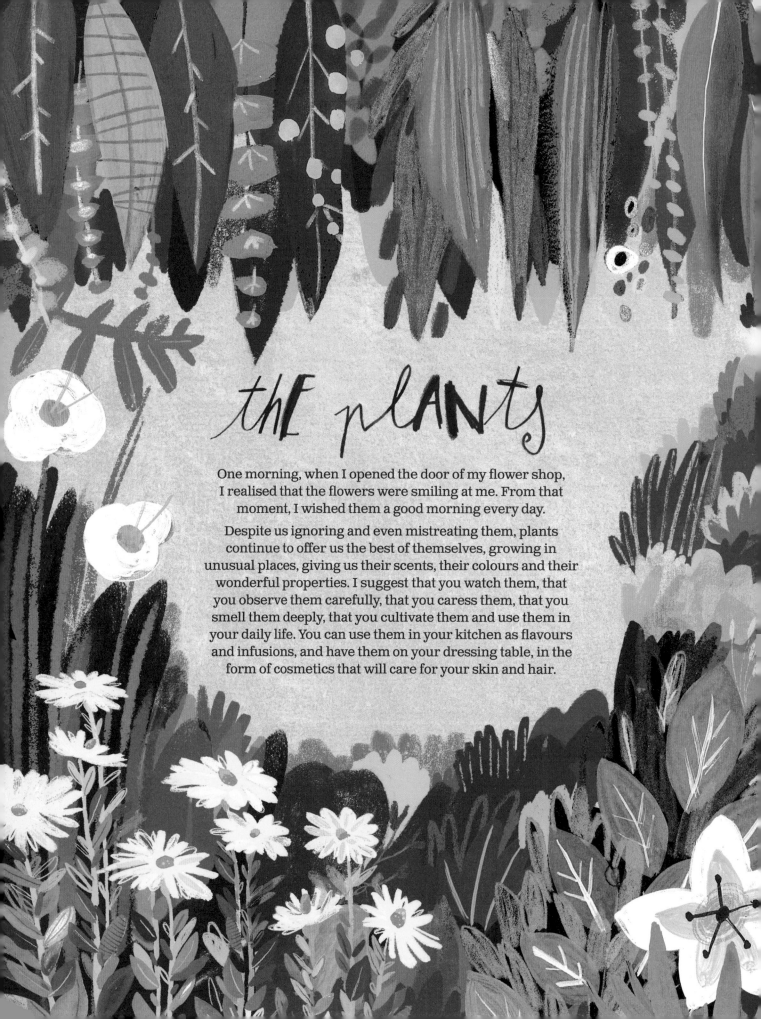

# the plants

One morning, when I opened the door of my flower shop, I realised that the flowers were smiling at me. From that moment, I wished them a good morning every day.

Despite us ignoring and even mistreating them, plants continue to offer us the best of themselves, growing in unusual places, giving us their scents, their colours and their wonderful properties. I suggest that you watch them, that you observe them carefully, that you caress them, that you smell them deeply, that you cultivate them and use them in your daily life. You can use them in your kitchen as flavours and infusions, and have them on your dressing table, in the form of cosmetics that will care for your skin and hair.

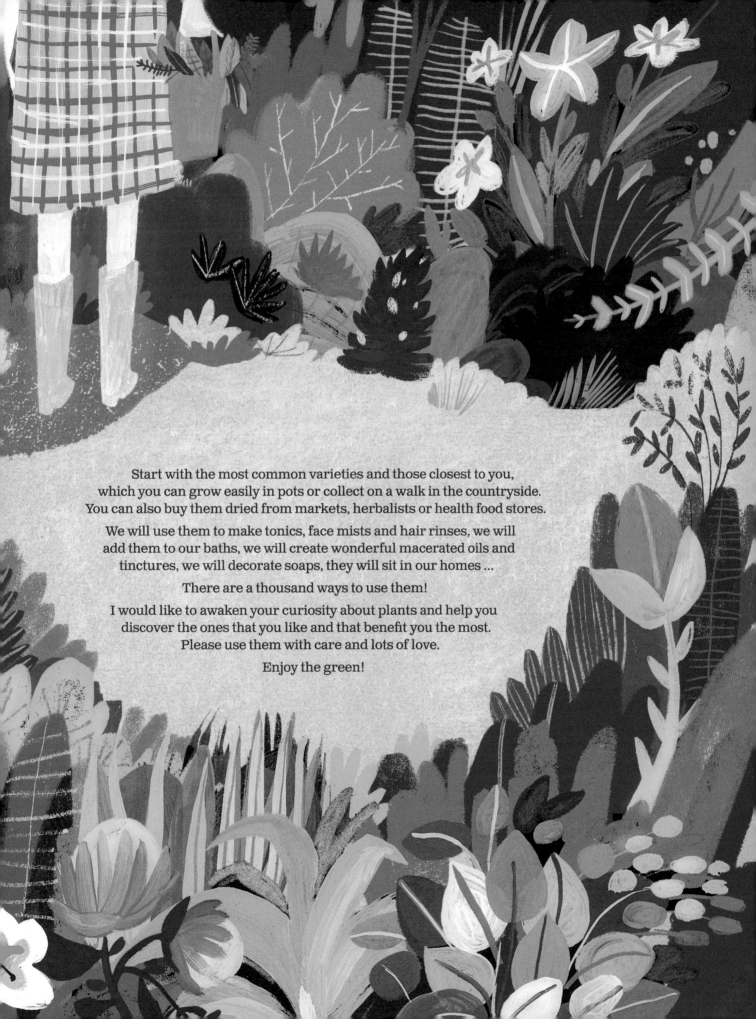

Start with the most common varieties and those closest to you,
which you can grow easily in pots or collect on a walk in the countryside.
You can also buy them dried from markets, herbalists or health food stores.

We will use them to make tonics, face mists and hair rinses, we will
add them to our baths, we will create wonderful macerated oils and
tinctures, we will decorate soaps, they will sit in our homes …

There are a thousand ways to use them!

I would like to awaken your curiosity about plants and help you
discover the ones that you like and that benefit you the most.
Please use them with care and lots of love.

Enjoy the green!

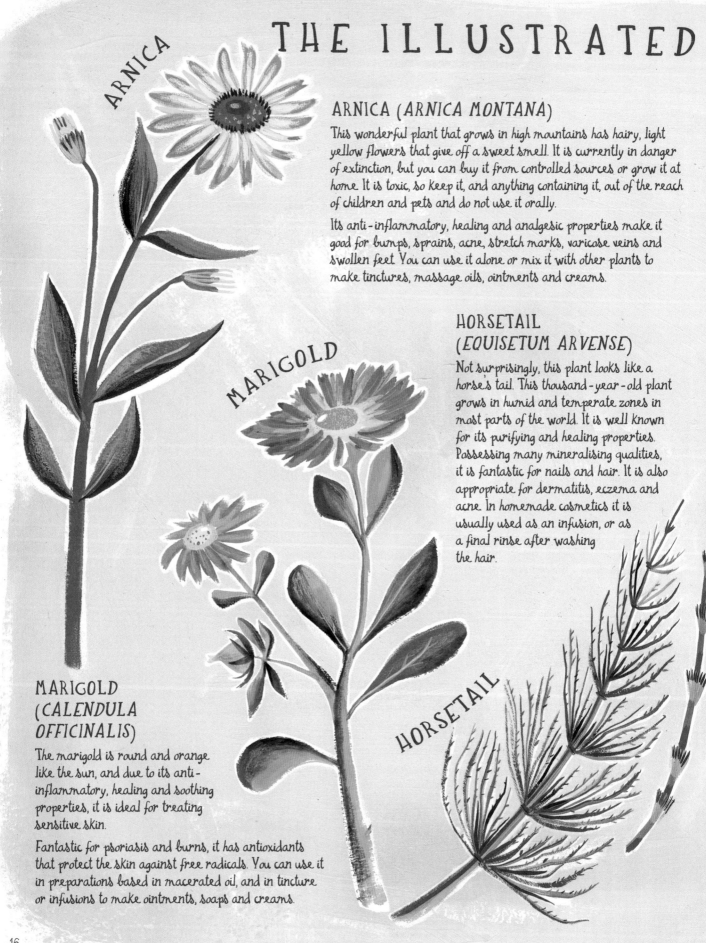

**ARNICA**

## ARNICA (ARNICA MONTANA)

This wonderful plant that grows in high mountains has hairy, light yellow flowers that give off a sweet smell. It is currently in danger of extinction, but you can buy it from controlled sources or grow it at home. It is toxic, so keep it, and anything containing it, out of the reach of children and pets and do not use it orally.

Its anti-inflammatory, healing and analgesic properties make it good for bumps, sprains, acne, stretch marks, varicose veins and swollen feet. You can use it alone or mix it with other plants to make tinctures, massage oils, ointments and creams.

## HORSETAIL (EQUISETUM ARVENSE)

Not surprisingly, this plant looks like a horse's tail. This thousand-year-old plant grows in humid and temperate zones in most parts of the world. It is well known for its purifying and healing properties. Possessing many mineralising qualities, it is fantastic for nails and hair. It is also appropriate for dermatitis, eczema and acne. In homemade cosmetics it is usually used as an infusion, or as a final rinse after washing the hair.

**MARIGOLD**

## MARIGOLD (CALENDULA OFFICINALIS)

The marigold is round and orange like the sun, and due to its anti-inflammatory, healing and soothing properties, it is ideal for treating sensitive skin.

Fantastic for psoriasis and burns, it has antioxidants that protect the skin against free radicals. You can use it in preparations based in macerated oil, and in tincture or infusions to make ointments, soaps and creams.

**HORSETAIL**

# HERBARIUM (I)

## BLUE GUM

## ALOE VERA

## ECHINACEA

## ALOE VERA (ALOE VERA)

Also simply called aloe, aloe vera is a type of cactus that grows in dry climates and contains a lot of cosmetic properties. We use the gelatinous-looking pulp of its leaves, which you can buy in health food stores or easily extract from the plant itself (use the oldest leaves).

Containing many nutrients, it has regenerating, astringent, soothing and healing properties. You can use it pure or in preparations such as masks, creams and soaps for the face, body and hair. It is ideal for soothing the skin after sun exposure and hair removal.

## BLUE GUM (EUCALYPTUS GLOBULUS)

This Australian tree is known for its medicinal properties, and is often used to treat respiratory tract diseases. Blue gum is antiseptic, antiviral and astringent.

In cosmetics we use it to regulate hair and skin fat, and to help with oral hygiene. It is usually used in macerated oils and infusions, and as an essential oil.

## ECHINACEA (ECHINACEA ANGUSTIFOLIA)

This plant of American origin is well known for its ability to increase the body's defences against infection (when taken orally) but it is also widely used in cosmetics as a regenerant, for anti-aging and in oral hygiene. You can prepare it as an infusion, a tincture or a macerated oil.

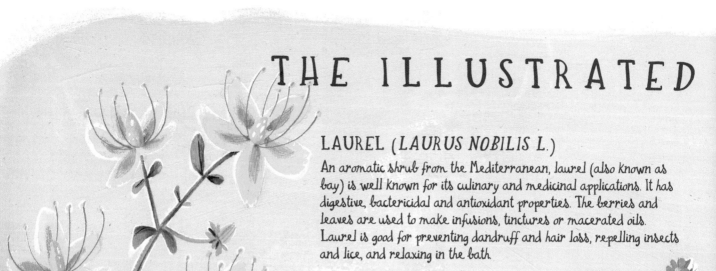

## LAUREL (*LAURUS NOBILIS L.*)

An aromatic shrub from the Mediterranean, laurel (also known as bay) is well known for its culinary and medicinal applications. It has digestive, bactericidal and antioxidant properties. The berries and leaves are used to make infusions, tinctures or macerated oils. Laurel is good for preventing dandruff and hair loss, repelling insects and lice, and relaxing in the bath.

## ST JOHN'S WORT (*HYPERICUM PERFORATUM*)

This plant has antidepressant and anti-anxiety effects. In cosmetics, we use it to regenerate the skin, and to treat bumps, wounds, sprains, muscle spasms and insect bites.

You can prepare it in tinctures, macerated oils and ointments. It must be used at night, as it is photosensitising.

## ST JOHN'S WORT

## PLANTAIN (*PLANTAGO MAJOR*)

Plantain is an edible plant used to treat respiratory and digestive conditions.

In cosmetics, it is known for its many regenerative and healing properties, in creams, tinctures and macerated oils. It is also prepared as an infusion to soothe tired eyes.

## PLANTAIN

## THYME

## THYME (*THYMUS VULGARIS*)

Widely used in Ancient Egypt and Greece, thyme is an aromatic seasoning plant common in Mediterranean cuisine. It has disinfectant and digestive properties, and is usually taken as an infusion to help treat colds, angina, bronchitis, indigestion, flatulence and colic.

In topical form, it is recommended for acne, as it is a sebaceous regulator and disinfectant. It has regenerative and healing properties, and is very common in hair lotions, creams, oils and ointments.

# HERBARIUM (II)

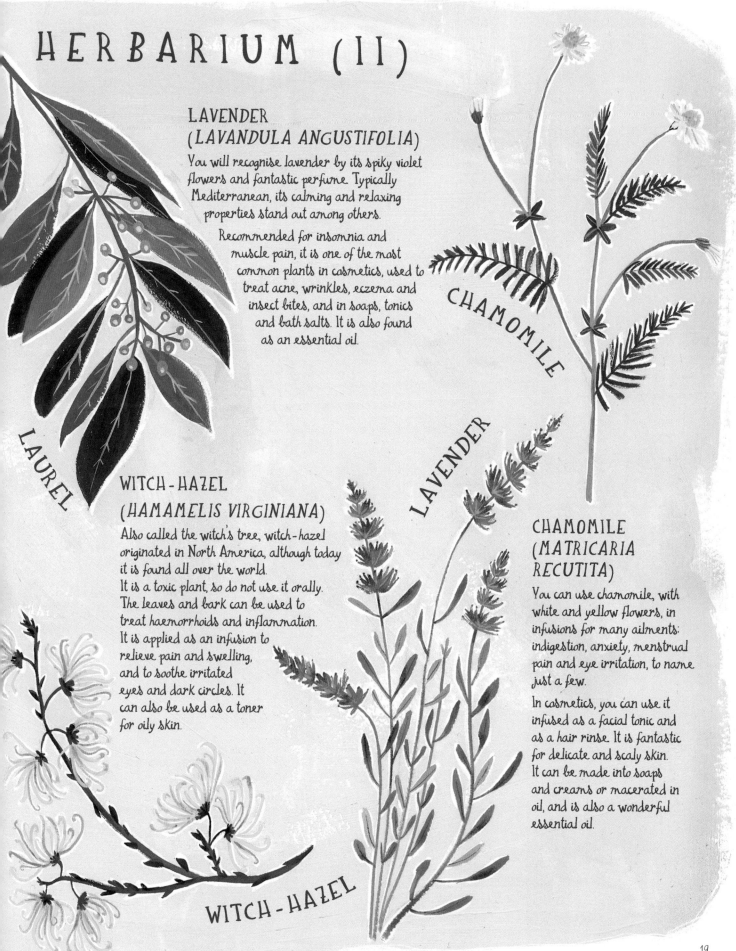

### LAVENDER
### (LAVANDULA ANGUSTIFOLIA)

You will recognise lavender by its spiky violet flowers and fantastic perfume. Typically Mediterranean, its calming and relaxing properties stand out among others.

Recommended for insomnia and muscle pain, it is one of the most common plants in cosmetics, used to treat acne, wrinkles, eczema and insect bites, and in soaps, tonics and bath salts. It is also found as an essential oil.

CHAMOMILE

LAUREL

### WITCH-HAZEL
### (HAMAMELIS VIRGINIANA)

Also called the witch's tree, witch-hazel originated in North America, although today it is found all over the world.
It is a toxic plant, so do not use it orally. The leaves and bark can be used to treat haemorrhoids and inflammation. It is applied as an infusion to relieve pain and swelling, and to soothe irritated eyes and dark circles. It can also be used as a toner for oily skin.

LAVENDER

### CHAMOMILE
### (MATRICARIA RECUTITA)

You can use chamomile, with white and yellow flowers, in infusions for many ailments: indigestion, anxiety, menstrual pain and eye irritation, to name just a few.

In cosmetics, you can use it infused as a facial tonic and as a hair rinse. It is fantastic for delicate and scaly skin. It can be made into soaps and creams or macerated in oil, and is also a wonderful essential oil.

WITCH-HAZEL

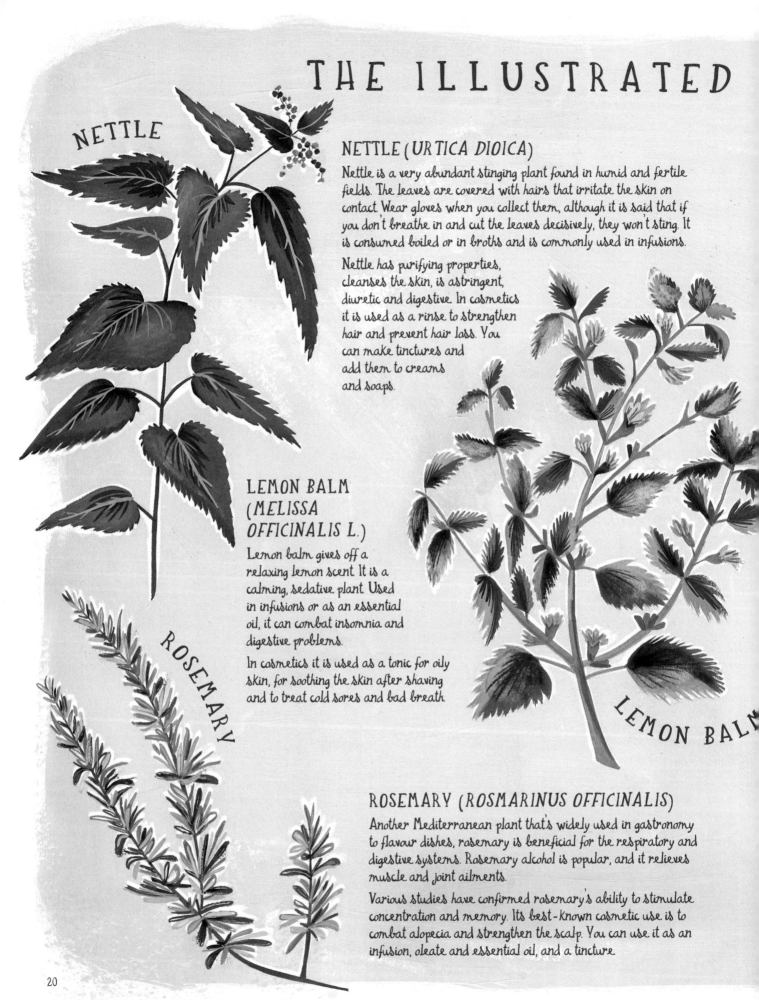

NETTLE

## NETTLE (*URTICA DIOICA*)

Nettle is a very abundant stinging plant found in humid and fertile fields. The leaves are covered with hairs that irritate the skin on contact. Wear gloves when you collect them, although it is said that if you don't breathe in and cut the leaves decisively, they won't sting. It is consumed boiled or in broths and is commonly used in infusions.

Nettle has purifying properties, cleanses the skin, is astringent, diuretic and digestive. In cosmetics it is used as a rinse to strengthen hair and prevent hair loss. You can make tinctures and add them to creams and soaps.

## LEMON BALM (*MELISSA OFFICINALIS L.*)

Lemon balm gives off a relaxing lemon scent. It is a calming, sedative plant. Used in infusions or as an essential oil, it can combat insomnia and digestive problems.

In cosmetics it is used as a tonic for oily skin, for soothing the skin after shaving and to treat cold sores and bad breath.

ROSEMARY

LEMON BALM

## ROSEMARY (*ROSMARINUS OFFICINALIS*)

Another Mediterranean plant that's widely used in gastronomy to flavour dishes, rosemary is beneficial for the respiratory and digestive systems. Rosemary alcohol is popular, and it relieves muscle and joint ailments.

Various studies have confirmed rosemary's ability to stimulate concentration and memory. Its best-known cosmetic use is to combat alopecia and strengthen the scalp. You can use it as an infusion, oleate and essential oil, and a tincture.

# HERBARIUM (III)

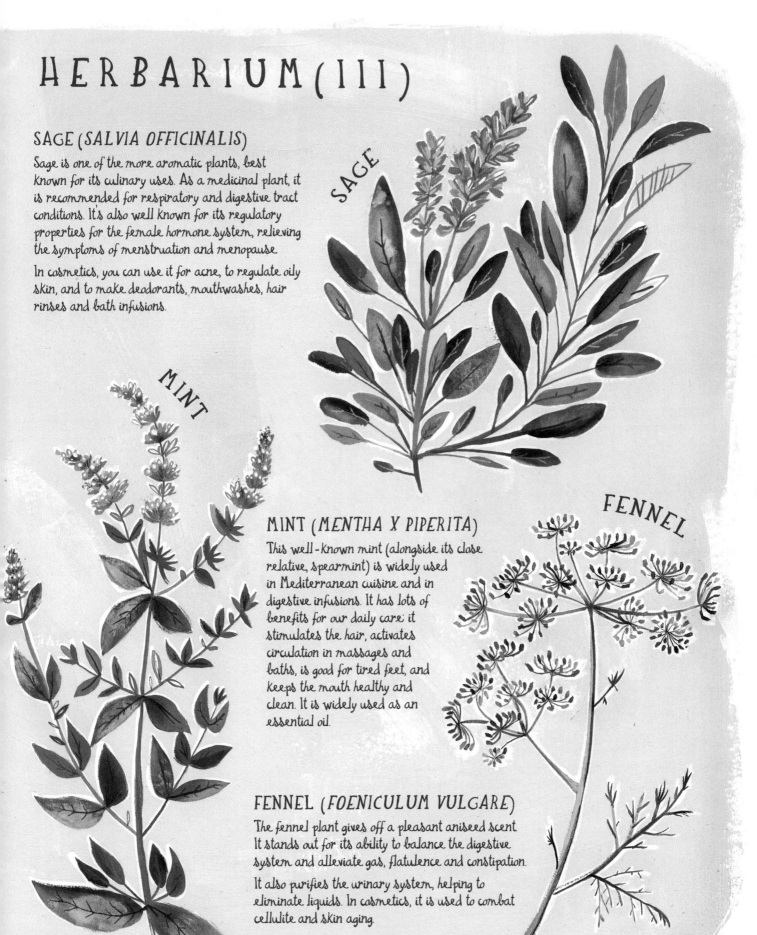

## SAGE (SALVIA OFFICINALIS)

Sage is one of the more aromatic plants, best known for its culinary uses. As a medicinal plant, it is recommended for respiratory and digestive tract conditions. It's also well known for its regulatory properties for the female hormone system, relieving the symptoms of menstruation and menopause.

In cosmetics, you can use it for acne, to regulate oily skin, and to make deodorants, mouthwashes, hair rinses and bath infusions.

## MINT (MENTHA X PIPERITA)

This well-known mint (alongside its close relative, spearmint) is widely used in Mediterranean cuisine and in digestive infusions. It has lots of benefits for our daily care: it stimulates the hair, activates circulation in massages and baths, is good for tired feet, and keeps the mouth healthy and clean. It is widely used as an essential oil.

## FENNEL (FOENICULUM VULGARE)

The fennel plant gives off a pleasant aniseed scent. It stands out for its ability to balance the digestive system and alleviate gas, flatulence and constipation.

It also purifies the urinary system, helping to eliminate liquids. In cosmetics, it is used to combat cellulite and skin aging.

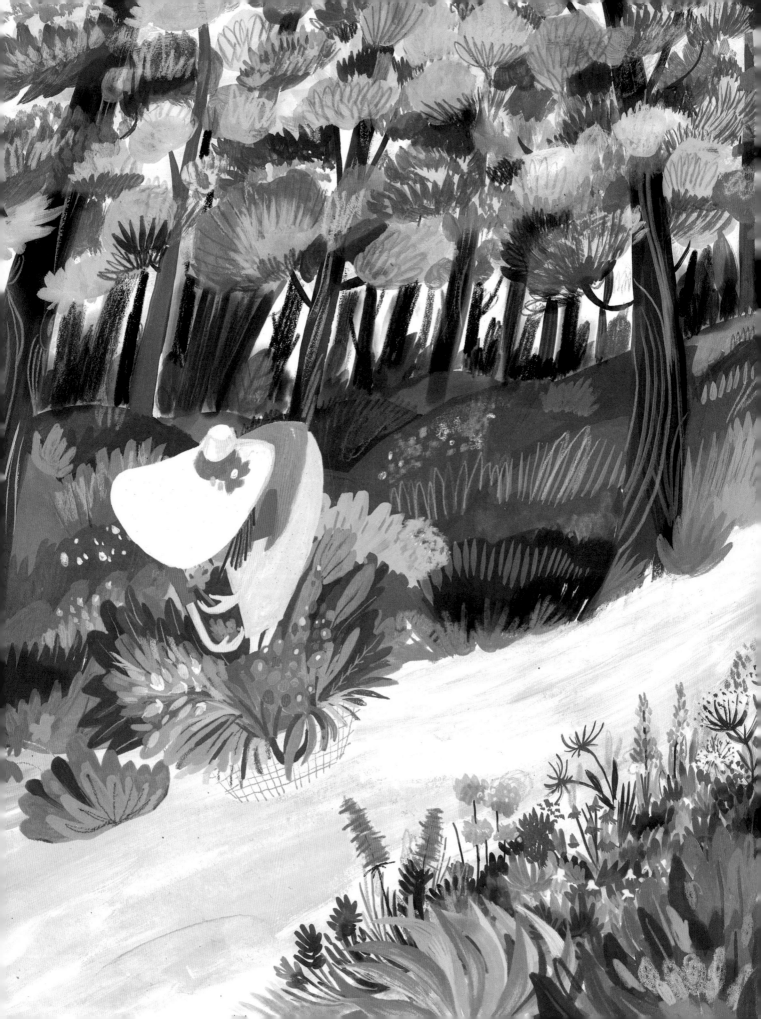

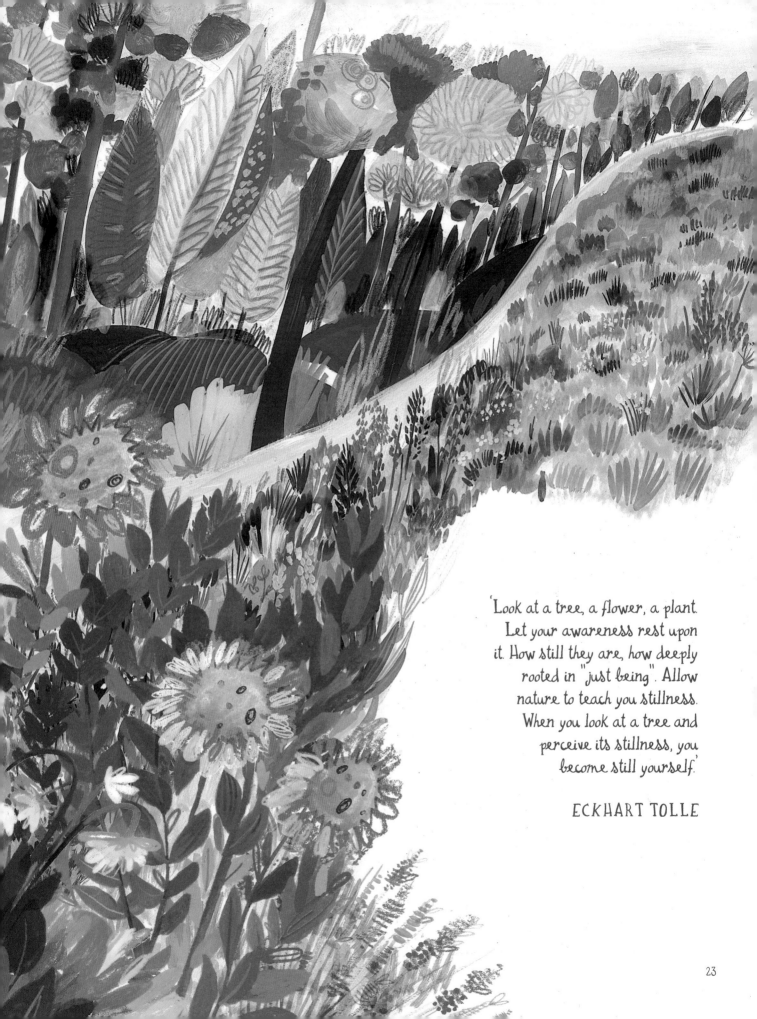

'Look at a tree, a flower, a plant.
Let your awareness rest upon
it. How still they are, how deeply
rooted in "just being". Allow
nature to teach you stillness.
When you look at a tree and
perceive its stillness, you
become still yourself.'

ECKHART TOLLE

# COLLECTION AND PRESERVATION

IF YOU HAVE A SMALL BALCONY OR YOU LIKE TO WALK IN THE COUNTRYSIDE,
YOU CAN GROW OR COLLECT FRESH PLANTS AND MAKE YOUR COSMETICS WITH THEM.
THE BEST WAY TO PRESERVE THEM IS AIR DRYING, OR IF YOU PREFER, YOU CAN BUY
THEM DRIED FROM HEALTH FOOD STORES OR MARKETS.

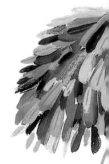

## COLLECTION KIT

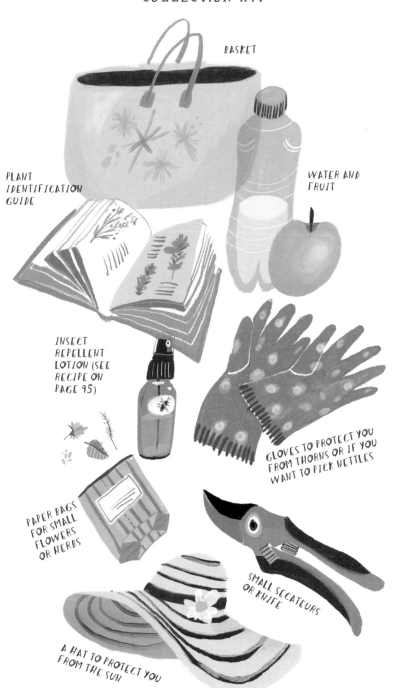

BASKET

WATER AND FRUIT

PLANT IDENTIFICATION GUIDE

INSECT REPELLENT LOTION (SEE RECIPE ON PAGE 95)

GLOVES TO PROTECT YOU FROM THORNS OR IF YOU WANT TO PICK NETTLES

PAPER BAGS FOR SMALL FLOWERS OR HERBS

SMALL SECATEURS OR KNIFE

A HAT TO PROTECT YOU FROM THE SUN

## HARVESTING

If you gather plants yourself in the wild, use a reliable guide to help you identify them. Make sure they are not toxic or in danger of extinction and if in doubt, leave them behind.

It is important to harvest when the plants are full of active ingredients, which is usually just before they are flowering. If you just want to harvest the flowers, wait for the plant to be in full bloom.

Plants must be free of pesticides, insects and dirt, so the best ones to use are those away from roads or factories. Choose vigorous and strong specimens. The best time of the day to harvest is in the morning, right after the dew lifts. Avoid harvesting in full sun, or when it's raining or foggy.

Do not take the entire plant or all of its flowers. Collect only what you need. Make a clean cut using small, sharp secateurs or a knife, taking care not to tear or damage the stem. Use a cloth bag or a basket to carry what you have collected, not a plastic bag. You can enhance your excursion by stopping to draw the plants that you are collecting or the ones that attract your attention.

Breathe and enjoy!

LAVENDER, ROSEMARY, THYME, MINT AND SAGE ARE JUST SOME OF THE PLANTS YOU CAN EASILY GROW FROM SEED AT HOME. YOU CAN ALSO BUY THEM AS GROWN PLANTS (BEWARE OF PESTICIDES) OR GERMINATE SEEDS AND TRANSFER THEM INTO BIGGER POTS.

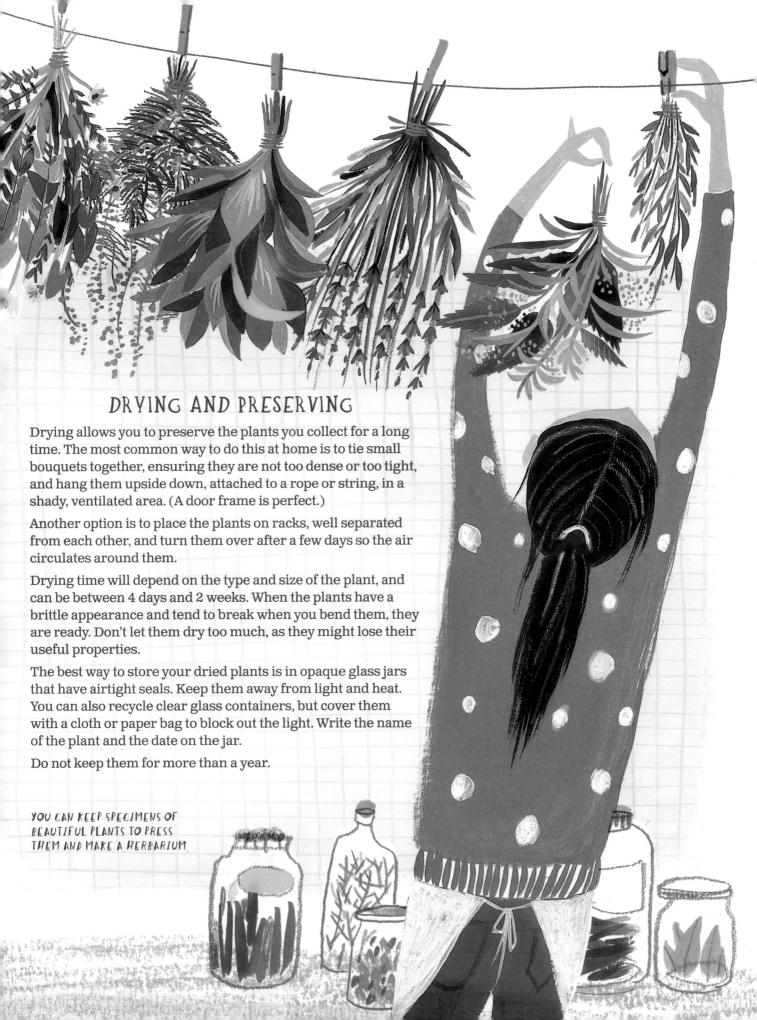

# DRYING AND PRESERVING

Drying allows you to preserve the plants you collect for a long time. The most common way to do this at home is to tie small bouquets together, ensuring they are not too dense or too tight, and hang them upside down, attached to a rope or string, in a shady, ventilated area. (A door frame is perfect.)

Another option is to place the plants on racks, well separated from each other, and turn them over after a few days so the air circulates around them.

Drying time will depend on the type and size of the plant, and can be between 4 days and 2 weeks. When the plants have a brittle appearance and tend to break when you bend them, they are ready. Don't let them dry too much, as they might lose their useful properties.

The best way to store your dried plants is in opaque glass jars that have airtight seals. Keep them away from light and heat. You can also recycle clear glass containers, but cover them with a cloth or paper bag to block out the light. Write the name of the plant and the date on the jar.

Do not keep them for more than a year.

YOU CAN KEEP SPECIMENS OF BEAUTIFUL PLANTS TO PRESS THEM AND MAKE A HERBARIUM.

# PLANT PREPARATIONS (1)

THERE ARE SEVERAL WAYS TO HARNESS THE POWERFUL BENEFITS OF YOUR PLANTS AND USE THEM INTERNALLY AND EXTERNALLY. THE AIM IS TO EXTRACT THE ACTIVE ELEMENTS TO MAKE YOUR OWN COSMETICS. HERE ARE SOME SIMPLE METHODS THAT YOU CAN USE AT HOME.

## USING DRY PLANTS

When your herbs are ready, you can use them in your personal hygiene in several ways:

- Add a handful of dried plants to your bath to help you relax. They also have disinfecting and cleansing properties. Put them in a small gauze bag to make it easier to remove them from the bathtub.

- Use them in facial steam baths to cleanse your pores, relax your skin and ease your breathing.

- Crush or shred them and use them in body scrubs for your feet, ankles, knees and elbows.

- Use them as an air freshener for your home or to decorate soaps.

## INFUSIONS

Infusions are the best known preparations and the easiest to prepare. Although they are usually intended for internal use, in cosmetics we also use infusions to make face and body tonics, hair rinses and masks, and poultices.

To make an infusion, bring some water to the boil then remove from the heat. Add the plant, then cover and leave to rest for 5 to 10 minutes.

If you want to increase the intensity of the infusion, extend the rest time.

Once it is cool, strain the liquid from the solids. The shelf life is relatively short – a maximum of 24 hours – and it must be kept refrigerated.

## DECOCTIONS

Decoction is the process of extracting the active ingredients from the hard parts of plants (such as barks and roots). It consists of heating water, adding the dry plant and bringing the mixture to the boil over a very gentle heat for between 3 and 15 minutes.

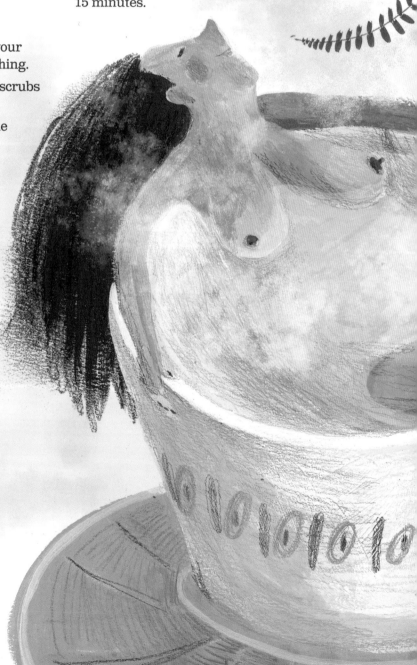

## TINCTURES

In tinctures, alcohol is used as a base element to preserve and extract the active ingredients of plants.

Place the plant into a sterilised glass jar and cover with a high-volume alcohol (40–45% ABV). Some people use vodka. An opaque jar is ideal, but you can also store a transparent jar in a closet or inside a paper or cloth bag so that it is not exposed to light.

Let the mixture rest for 28 days (a lunar cycle) then filter it through a gauze strainer or an unbleached coffee filter.

Given the high concentration of active ingredients, it is best to store tinctures in a sterilised bottle and use a dropper to properly measure quantities. Write the ingredients and the date on the bottle.

You can use tinctures in lotions, soaps and tonics. Be very careful if you use them undiluted, as the alcohol can irritate the skin.

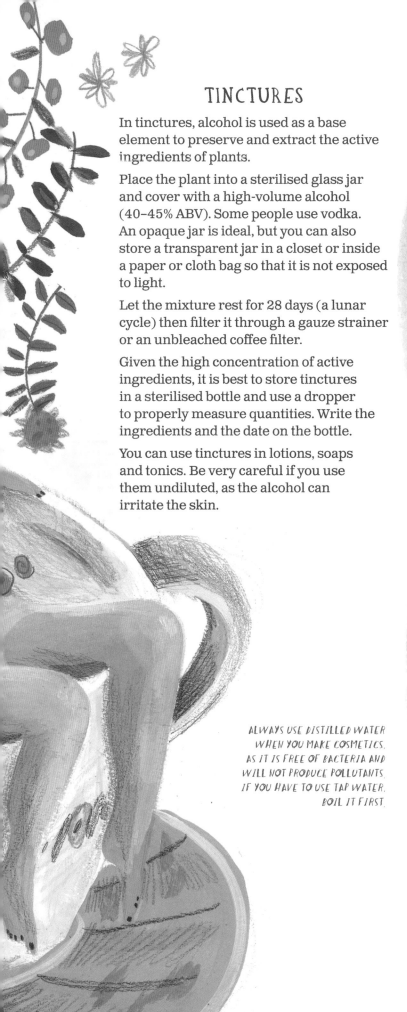

ALWAYS USE DISTILLED WATER WHEN YOU MAKE COSMETICS, AS IT IS FREE OF BACTERIA AND WILL NOT PRODUCE POLLUTANTS. IF YOU HAVE TO USE TAP WATER, BOIL IT FIRST.

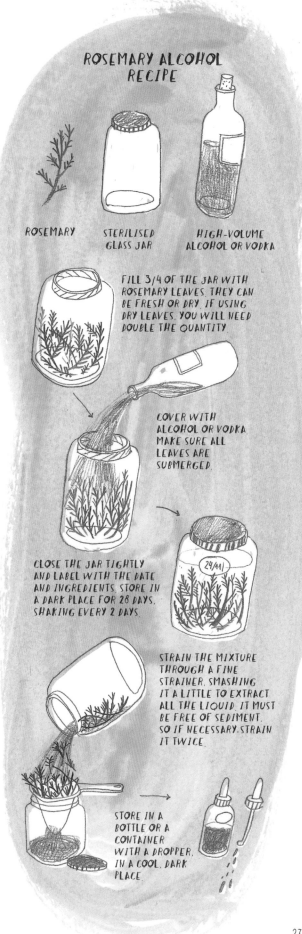

ROSEMARY ALCOHOL RECIPE

ROSEMARY

STERILISED GLASS JAR

HIGH-VOLUME ALCOHOL OR VODKA

FILL 3/4 OF THE JAR WITH ROSEMARY LEAVES. THEY CAN BE FRESH OR DRY. IF USING DRY LEAVES, YOU WILL NEED DOUBLE THE QUANTITY.

COVER WITH ALCOHOL OR VODKA. MAKE SURE ALL LEAVES ARE SUBMERGED.

CLOSE THE JAR TIGHTLY AND LABEL WITH THE DATE AND INGREDIENTS. STORE IN A DARK PLACE FOR 28 DAYS, SHAKING EVERY 2 DAYS.

STRAIN THE MIXTURE THROUGH A FINE STRAINER, SMASHING IT A LITTLE TO EXTRACT ALL THE LIQUID. IT MUST BE FREE OF SEDIMENT, SO IF NECESSARY, STRAIN IT TWICE.

STORE IN A BOTTLE OR A CONTAINER WITH A DROPPER, IN A COOL, DARK PLACE.

# PLANT PREPARATIONS (II)

## MACERATED OR INFUSED OILS

A GOOD VEGETABLE OIL IS A TREASURE. ENHANCE ITS PROPERTIES BY SOAKING PLANTS AND FLOWERS IN IT, LETTING THE POWER OF THE SUN AND THE MOON DO THE REST. YOU CAN USE IT TO MAKE WONDERFUL COSMETICS OR SIMPLY PUT IT STRAIGHT ONTO YOUR SKIN.

### MACERATIONS COMMONLY USED IN COSMETICS

Healing, restorative and soothing. Very aromatic and relaxing. For facial and body creams and massage oils.

Regenerative, especially for sensitive skin, dermatitis, inflammation and insect bites.

Soothing and regenerating. Especially good for delicate and baby skin, redness, allergies and peeling.

Anti-inflammatory and toning. Ideal for the scalp, and for making masks, shampoos and massage oils.

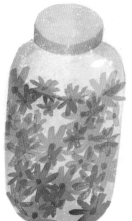

lavender

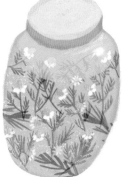

marigold

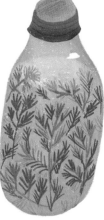

chamomile

rosemary

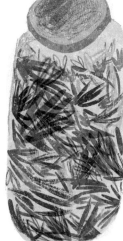

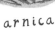
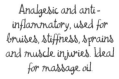

arnica

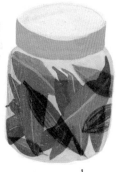

laurel

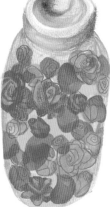

rose

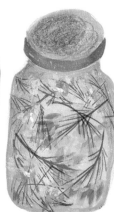

St John's wort

Analgesic and anti-inflammatory, used for bruises, stiffness, sprains and muscle injuries. Ideal for massage oil.

Disinfecting, antiseptic, fungicidal, healing and anti-inflammatory. Ideal for making soap, shampoo and body oil.

Anti-aging, regenerating and soothing. Ideal for mature skin.

Analgesic and healing agent for bumps and wounds. Astringent for oily skin. Photosensitiser, use at night.

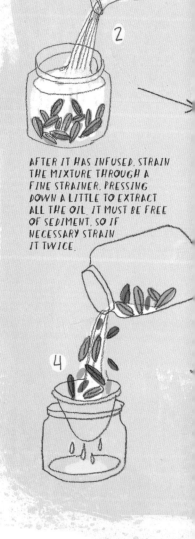

STEP-BY-STEP: MACERATED OIL

1

STERILISE A GLASS JAR AND ADD THE CHOPPED PLANTS.

ADD THE VEGETABLE OIL, ENSURING YOU COVER THE PLANTS FULLY.

2

AFTER IT HAS INFUSED, STRAIN THE MIXTURE THROUGH A FINE STRAINER, PRESSING DOWN A LITTLE TO EXTRACT ALL THE OIL. IT MUST BE FREE OF SEDIMENT, SO IF NECESSARY STRAIN IT TWICE.

4

# MACERATED 'IN SUN AND SERENITY'

This ancient practice allows plants to impart their properties into oil. The process consists of leaving the preparation in the open (in light, but not full sun, which could spoil it) so that it undergoes the gradual temperature changes of night and day. The usual period is 28 days (a lunar cycle) or 42 days.

*The sun and the moon will do the rest*

PUT A PIECE OF PLASTIC WRAP OVER THE OPENING BEFORE CLOSING THE JAR, TO SEAL IT AND PROTECT THE OIL FROM RUSTING ON THE LID.
PUT IT IN THE SUN AND SERENITY FOR 28 OR 42 DAYS. STIR THE MIXTURE DAILY.

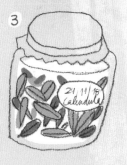

STORE IT IN A COOL, DARK PLACE. LABEL WITH THE DATE AND INGREDIENTS.

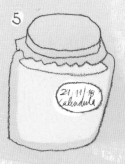

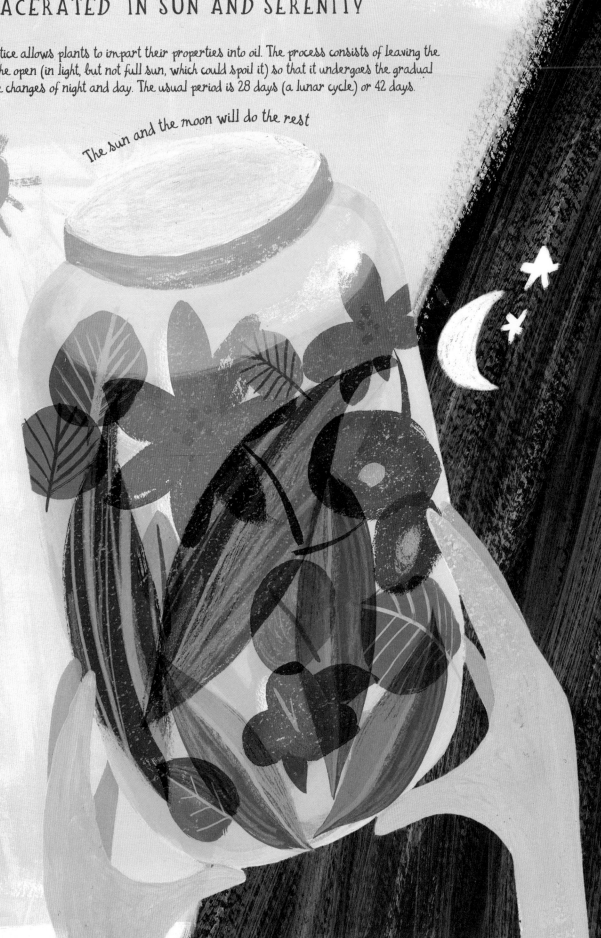

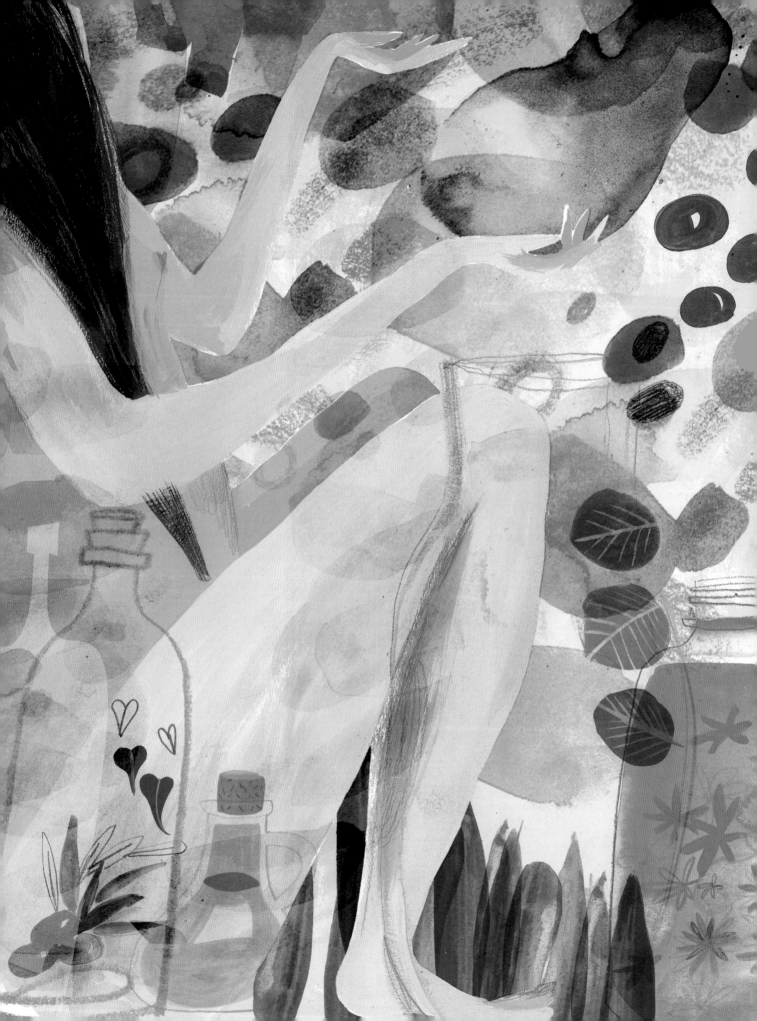

# vegetable oils and fats

Observing the colour and shine of oil on your skin is a magical experience. It looks like a ray of sunshine is running along your fingers. Rub the oil between your hands and watch how your skin absorbs it. I remember my mother rubbing her hands with olive oil and lemon after washing the dishes to hydrate and lighten them.

From dark oranges to greens and yellows, the colours (and smells) of vegetable oils vary according to their origin. These oils are extracted from seeds and other sources, like almond, argan or olive. Most of these oils are used in the kitchen and they have many beneficial properties, including, when used topically, for your skin.

Vegetable oils have long been a basic component in our daily beauty routines. They must be quality oils extracted by cold pressing, which guarantees that their properties are intact. It is also important that they are organically produced, without pesticides or fertilisers. I recommend purchasing from specialised stores or local suppliers.

They are moisturising, nourishing, regenerating and protective. They can be used as antioxidants and to soften your skin. But they are also a powerful cosmetic for the face, body, nails and hair, and their properties are multiplied if you infuse them with herbs (see pages 28–29) or add essential oils (pages 40–41 ). By mixing them with butters and waxes, you can get other textures, such as balms, ointments and creams.

Contrary to popular belief, they are also suitable for oily skin, as some have sebum-regulating qualities. It is important to know the properties of each kind of oil in order to use them properly.

Keep your oils in opaque jars, away from light, cold, humidity and heat. In the warmer months, you can store them in the fridge. To use them, warm them with your fingers before applying with gentle massage.

Enjoy the liquid gold that nourishes your skin.

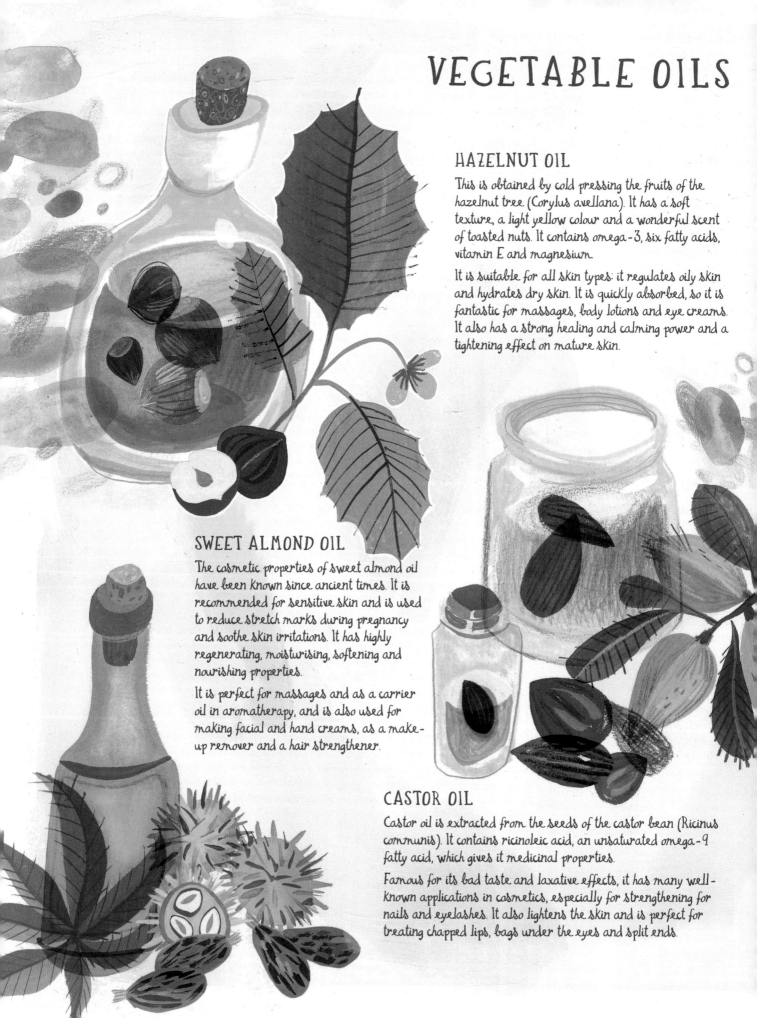

# VEGETABLE OILS

## HAZELNUT OIL

This is obtained by cold pressing the fruits of the hazelnut tree. (Corylus avellana). It has a soft texture, a light yellow colour and a wonderful scent of toasted nuts. It contains omega-3, six fatty acids, vitamin E and magnesium.

It is suitable for all skin types: it regulates oily skin and hydrates dry skin. It is quickly absorbed, so it is fantastic for massages, body lotions and eye creams. It also has a strong healing and calming power and a tightening effect on mature skin.

## SWEET ALMOND OIL

The cosmetic properties of sweet almond oil have been known since ancient times. It is recommended for sensitive skin and is used to reduce stretch marks during pregnancy and soothe skin irritations. It has highly regenerating, moisturising, softening and nourishing properties.

It is perfect for massages and as a carrier oil in aromatherapy, and is also used for making facial and hand creams, as a make-up remover and a hair strengthener.

## CASTOR OIL

Castor oil is extracted from the seeds of the castor bean (Ricinus communis). It contains ricinoleic acid, an unsaturated omega-9 fatty acid, which gives it medicinal properties.

Famous for its bad taste and laxative effects, it has many well-known applications in cosmetics, especially for strengthening for nails and eyelashes. It also lightens the skin and is perfect for treating chapped lips, bags under the eyes and split ends.

# IN COSMETICS (I)

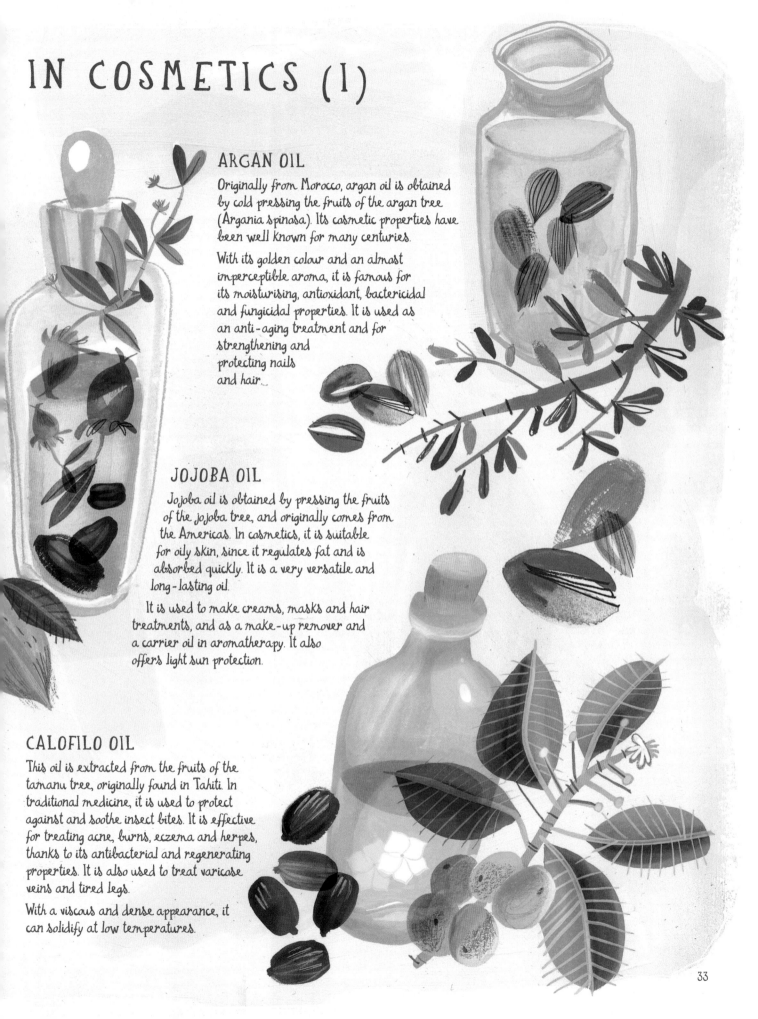

### ARGAN OIL

Originally from Morocco, argan oil is obtained by cold pressing the fruits of the argan tree (Argania spinosa). Its cosmetic properties have been well known for many centuries.

With its golden colour and an almost imperceptible aroma, it is famous for its moisturising, antioxidant, bactericidal and fungicidal properties. It is used as an anti-aging treatment and for strengthening and protecting nails and hair.

### JOJOBA OIL

Jojoba oil is obtained by pressing the fruits of the jojoba tree, and originally comes from the Americas. In cosmetics, it is suitable for oily skin, since it regulates fat and is absorbed quickly. It is a very versatile and long-lasting oil.

It is used to make creams, masks and hair treatments, and as a make-up remover and a carrier oil in aromatherapy. It also offers light sun protection.

### CALOFILO OIL

This oil is extracted from the fruits of the tamanu tree, originally found in Tahiti. In traditional medicine, it is used to protect against and soothe insect bites. It is effective for treating acne, burns, eczema and herpes, thanks to its antibacterial and regenerating properties. It is also used to treat varicose veins and tired legs.

With a viscous and dense appearance, it can solidify at low temperatures.

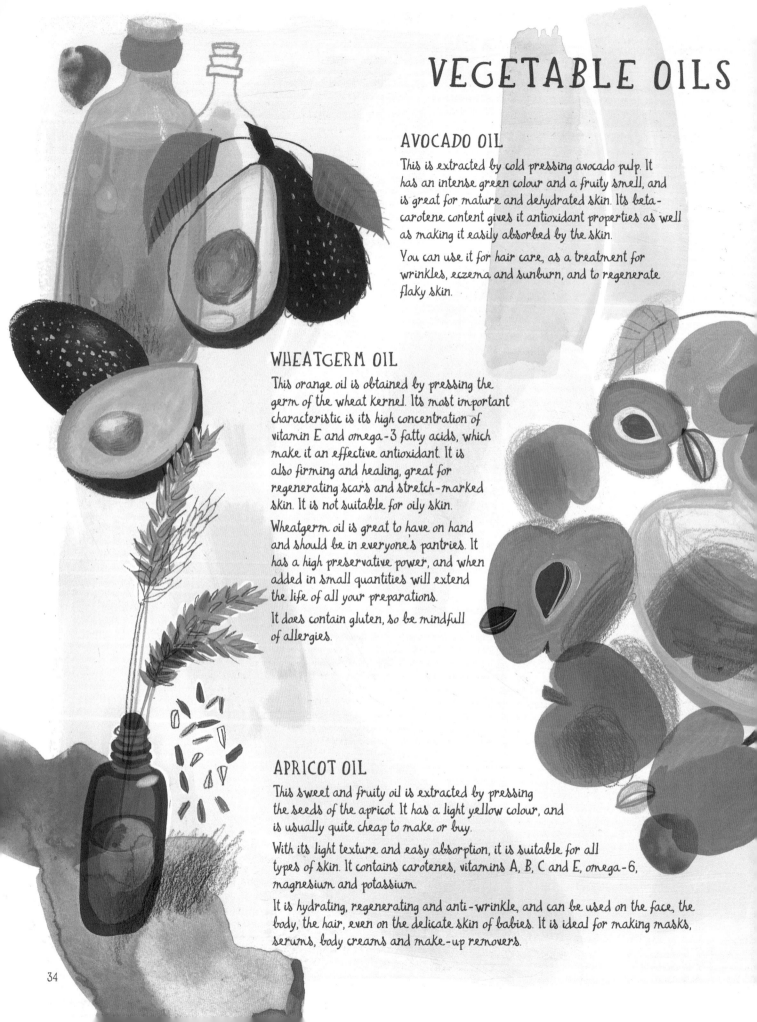

# VEGETABLE OILS

## AVOCADO OIL

This is extracted by cold pressing avocado pulp. It has an intense green colour and a fruity smell, and is great for mature and dehydrated skin. Its beta-carotene content gives it antioxidant properties as well as making it easily absorbed by the skin.

You can use it for hair care, as a treatment for wrinkles, eczema and sunburn, and to regenerate flaky skin.

## WHEATGERM OIL

This orange oil is obtained by pressing the germ of the wheat kernel. Its most important characteristic is its high concentration of vitamin E and omega-3 fatty acids, which make it an effective antioxidant. It is also firming and healing, great for regenerating scars and stretch-marked skin. It is not suitable for oily skin.

Wheatgerm oil is great to have on hand and should be in everyone's pantries. It has a high preservative power, and when added in small quantities will extend the life of all your preparations.

It does contain gluten, so be mindfull of allergies.

## APRICOT OIL

This sweet and fruity oil is extracted by pressing the seeds of the apricot. It has a light yellow colour, and is usually quite cheap to make or buy.

With its light texture and easy absorption, it is suitable for all types of skin. It contains carotenes, vitamins A, B, C and E, omega-6, magnesium and potassium.

It is hydrating, regenerating and anti-wrinkle, and can be used on the face, the body, the hair, even on the delicate skin of babies. It is ideal for making masks, serums, body creams and make-up removers.

# IN COSMETICS (II)

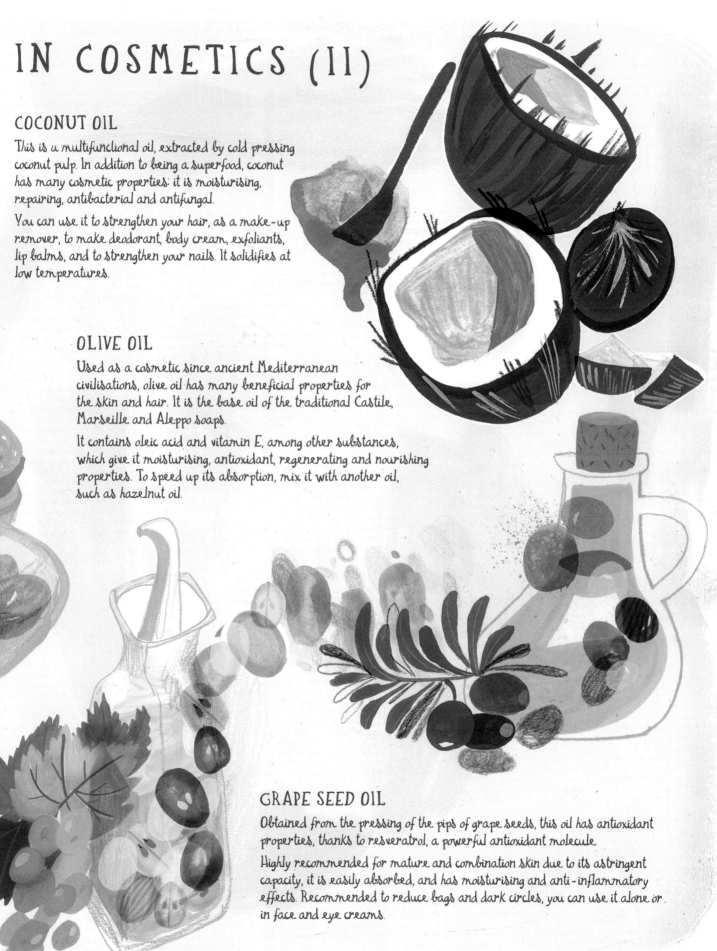

## COCONUT OIL

This is a multifunctional oil, extracted by cold pressing coconut pulp. In addition to being a superfood, coconut has many cosmetic properties: it is moisturising, repairing, antibacterial and antifungal.

You can use it to strengthen your hair, as a make-up remover, to make deodorant, body cream, exfoliants, lip balms, and to strengthen your nails. It solidifies at low temperatures.

## OLIVE OIL

Used as a cosmetic since ancient Mediterranean civilisations, olive oil has many beneficial properties for the skin and hair. It is the base oil of the traditional Castile, Marseille and Aleppo soaps.

It contains oleic acid and vitamin E, among other substances, which give it moisturising, antioxidant, regenerating and nourishing properties. To speed up its absorption, mix it with another oil, such as hazelnut oil.

## GRAPE SEED OIL

Obtained from the pressing of the pips of grape seeds, this oil has antioxidant properties, thanks to resveratrol, a powerful antioxidant molecule.

Highly recommended for mature and combination skin due to its astringent capacity, it is easily absorbed, and has moisturising and anti-inflammatory effects. Recommended to reduce bags and dark circles, you can use it alone or in face and eye creams.

## BORAGE OIL

Borage is known for its culinary use, as well as its regulatory effect on the female hormonal system. The oil is extracted by pressing the seeds of the plant.

In cosmetics, it is favoured for its moisturising and anti-inflammatory properties, and its absorption capacity. Borage oil is best used in combination with other oils or butters.

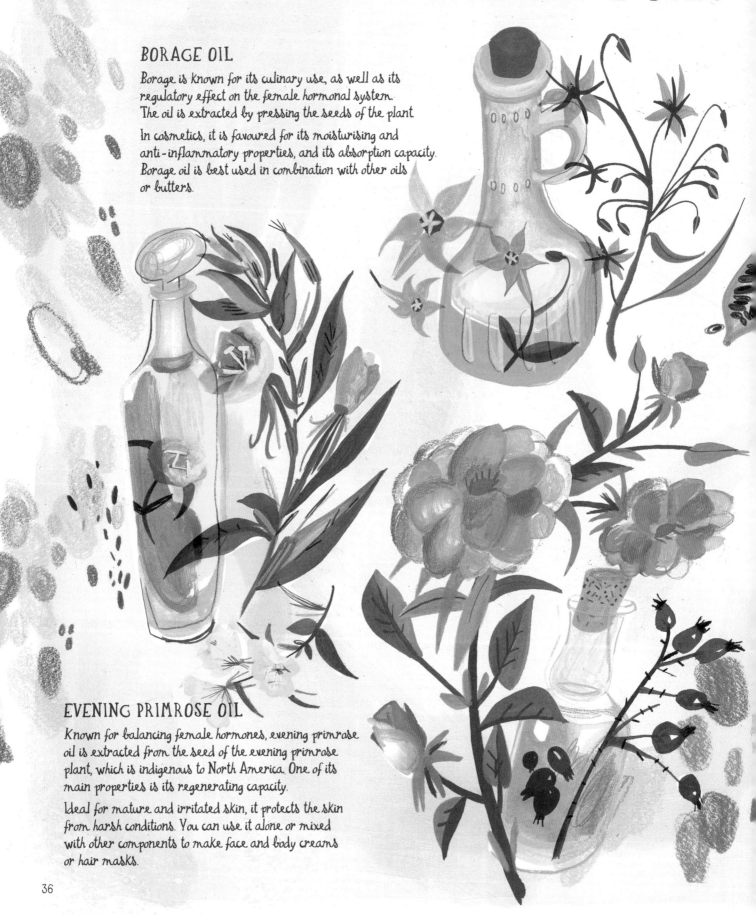

## EVENING PRIMROSE OIL

Known for balancing female hormones, evening primrose oil is extracted from the seed of the evening primrose plant, which is indigenous to North America. One of its main properties is its regenerating capacity.

Ideal for mature and irritated skin, it protects the skin from harsh conditions. You can use it alone or mixed with other components to make face and body creams or hair masks.

# IN COSMETICS (III)

## SUNFLOWER OIL

This well-known oil that is often found in kitchens also has great benefits for your skin.

With a light texture and an almost imperceptible smell, it is good as a regulator for acne-prone skin, a moisturiser for all skin types and a soothing agent for red or scaly skin. You can use it in creams, body lotions, soaps, masks and scrubs.

## SESAME OIL

The oil from the small sesame seed is suitable for moisturising mature skin, soothing irritations and reducing wrinkles.

It is a long-lasting oil that may even have a slight natural sunscreen effect

It is ideal for creating face and body creams, hair masks, make-up remover and massage oil.

## ROSEHIP OIL

Rosehip is a wild shrub and this wonderful oil is extracted from the fruits. Its properties are infinite, although its great regenerative capacity stands out. It delays the signs of aging, reduces stretch marks, accelerates wound healing, helps eliminate stains and reduces inflammation.

Used alone, it is a true beauty serum, but you can add it to other oils or fats to make body creams and hair masks. Rosehip oil is photosensitive, and can produce unwanted pigmentation in your skin. Do not use it before sun exposure.

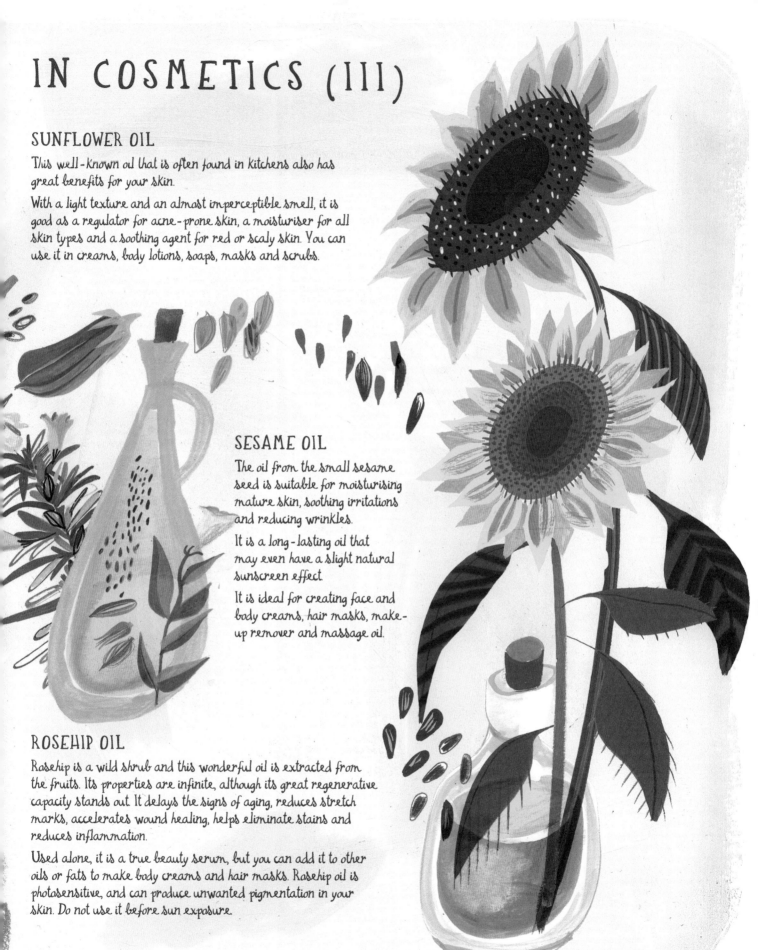

# VEGETABLE BUTTERS AND WAXES

BUTTERS, LIKE OILS, ARE VEGETABLE FATS THAT ARE EXTRACTED FROM FRUITS OR SEEDS.
THEY ARE VERY VALUABLE IN COSMETICS BECAUSE THEY HAVE MANY BENEFICIAL PROPERTIES FOR
THE SKIN AND HAIR. THEY ARE SOLID AT ROOM TEMPERATURE. THEIR COLOUR, SMELL AND TEXTURE
WILL VARY DEPENDING ON THEIR ORIGIN. THEY ARE IDEAL FOR MAKING CREAMS AND BALMS,
WHICH ARE OFTEN SOLID AND HAVE A RICH TEXTURE.

## SHEA BUTTER
## (BUTYROSPERMUM PARKII)

Shea butter is obtained from the nuts of the sacred
shea tree. Of African origin, it has been used
for centuries as food and to protect the skin and
hair. It is one of the most commonly used butters
in cosmetics.

It is important to ensure that its origin is
Fairtrade. There are many communities and
cooperatives of women in African nations who are
responsible for collecting it. It must be unrefined
so that it maintains all its properties. It is an
essential ingredient.

## COCOA BUTTER
## (THEOBROMA CACAO)

In addition to being a wonderful food, cocoa
butter offers essential cosmetic properties: it
is regenerative, protective and nourishing.

As well as having a fantastic chocolate
scent, it is high in vitamin E, which fights free
radicals and increases collagen production.
You can use it to make lip balms, and hand
and body creams.

## MANGO BUTTER
### (MANGIFERA INDICA)

Mango butter is extracted by cold pressing the stone that is inside the mango. It contains oils, vitamins and minerals, and offers light sun protection.

Quickly absorbed, it is soothing, moisturising, regenerating and an antioxidant. It also provides nutrients to the hair and repairs damaged ends. Ideal for balms and moisturising creams.

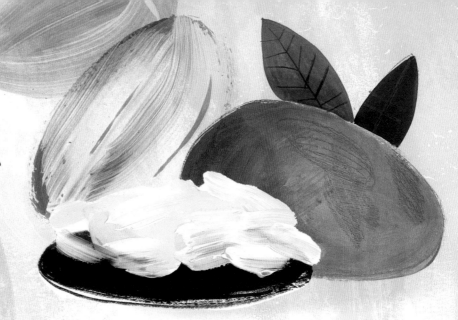

VEGETABLE WAXES ARE COMPLEX COMPOUNDS OF FATTY ACIDS, ALCOHOLS AND ESTERS. IN COSMETICS WE USE THEM AS EMULSIFIERS, AS THEY FACILITATE THE MIXING OF OIL AND WATER. IN ADDITION, THEY LEAVE A PROTECTIVE FILM ON THE SKIN, PROTECTING IT FROM DEHYDRATION.

## BEESWAX

This substance, secreted by bees to make their honeycombs, is extracted by heat. Rich in antioxidants and vitamin A, it protects and nourishes the skin and has anti-inflammatory and antioxidant properties.

You can use it to give regularity to creams, lip balms and eye contours, and to make depilatory creams.

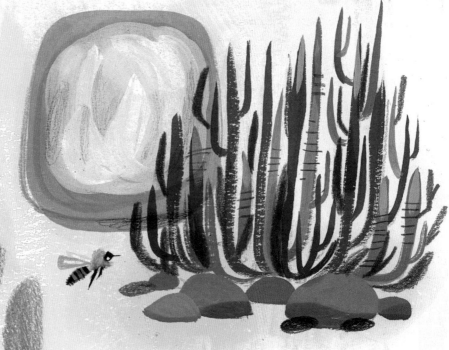

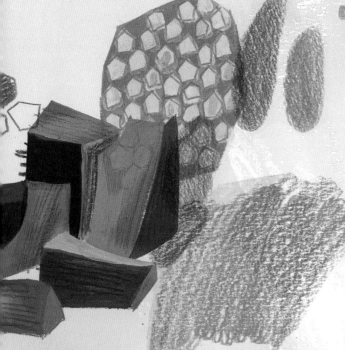

## CANDELILLA WAX
### (EUPHORBIA ANTISYPHILITICA)

Candelilla is a vegetable wax and a vegan alternative to beeswax. Its origin and use dates back to the indigenous people of northern Mexico, who used it for ornamental purposes.

It is extracted from the candelilla bush, which generates wax to protect itself from the environment and retain moisture. It has many uses in the chemical and food industries. In cosmetics it is used to give stability to creams and preparations, and for its moisturising and protective power.

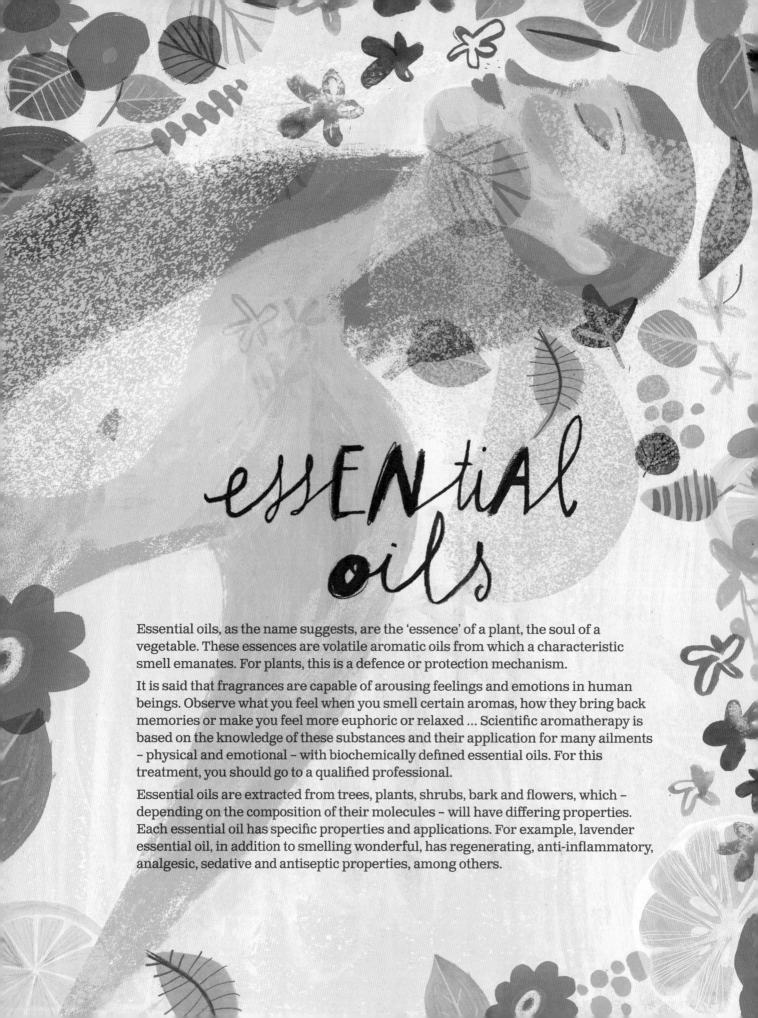

# essENtiAL oils

Essential oils, as the name suggests, are the 'essence' of a plant, the soul of a vegetable. These essences are volatile aromatic oils from which a characteristic smell emanates. For plants, this is a defence or protection mechanism.

It is said that fragrances are capable of arousing feelings and emotions in human beings. Observe what you feel when you smell certain aromas, how they bring back memories or make you feel more euphoric or relaxed ... Scientific aromatherapy is based on the knowledge of these substances and their application for many ailments – physical and emotional – with biochemically defined essential oils. For this treatment, you should go to a qualified professional.

Essential oils are extracted from trees, plants, shrubs, bark and flowers, which – depending on the composition of their molecules – will have differing properties. Each essential oil has specific properties and applications. For example, lavender essential oil, in addition to smelling wonderful, has regenerating, anti-inflammatory, analgesic, sedative and antiseptic properties, among others.

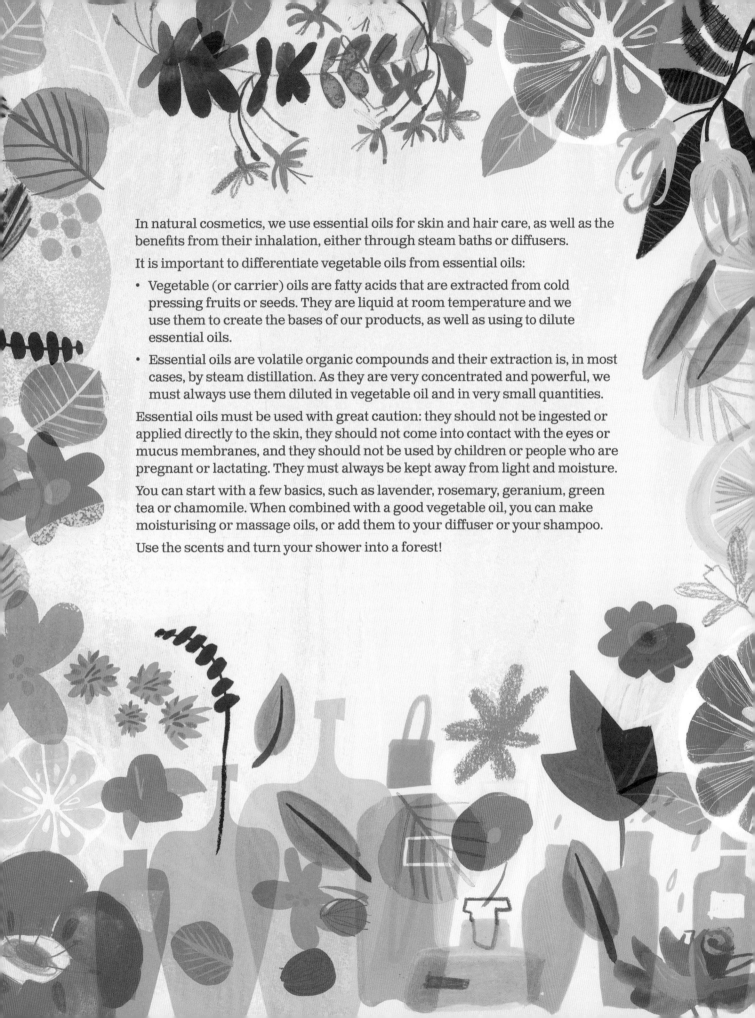

In natural cosmetics, we use essential oils for skin and hair care, as well as the benefits from their inhalation, either through steam baths or diffusers.

It is important to differentiate vegetable oils from essential oils:

- Vegetable (or carrier) oils are fatty acids that are extracted from cold pressing fruits or seeds. They are liquid at room temperature and we use them to create the bases of our products, as well as using to dilute essential oils.

- Essential oils are volatile organic compounds and their extraction is, in most cases, by steam distillation. As they are very concentrated and powerful, we must always use them diluted in vegetable oil and in very small quantities.

Essential oils must be used with great caution: they should not be ingested or applied directly to the skin, they should not come into contact with the eyes or mucus membranes, and they should not be used by children or people who are pregnant or lactating. They must always be kept away from light and moisture.

You can start with a few basics, such as lavender, rosemary, geranium, green tea or chamomile. When combined with a good vegetable oil, you can make moisturising or massage oils, or add them to your diffuser or your shampoo.

Use the scents and turn your shower into a forest!

# FLORAL ESSENTIAL OILS

WHEN WE SEE A FLOWER, WE INSTINCTIVELY MOVE CLOSER TO SMELL IT. THE SCENT TRANSPORTS US TO A GARDEN FULL OF LOVE AND WE OPEN OUR HEARTS. FLORAL ESSENTIAL OILS ARE USEFUL FOR COMBATING STRESS AND MENTAL FATIGUE, AND IN COSMETICS THEY ARE PRIZED FOR THEIR REGENERATIVE AND HEALING POWERS.

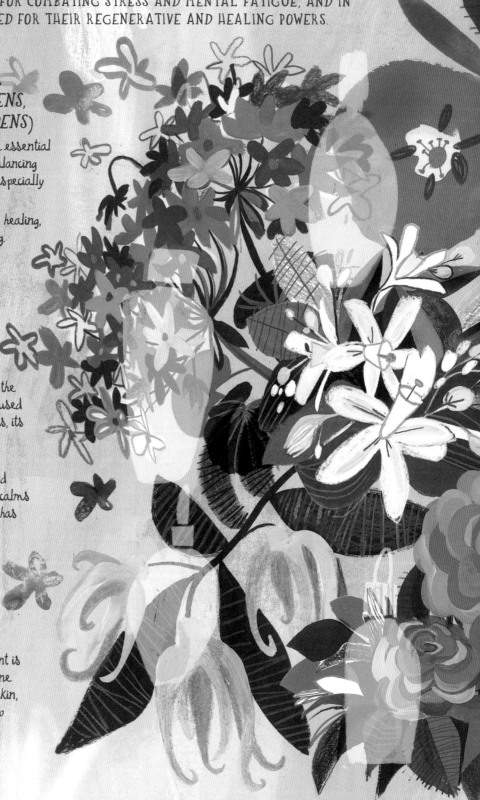

## GERANIUM ESSENTIAL OIL (PELARGONIUM GRAVEOLENS, P. ODORATISSIMUM, P. RADENS)

Often associated with the aroma of rose essential oil, geranium stands out for its great balancing power. It is suitable for all skin types, especially mixed, sensitive and acne-prone.

It is astringent, anti-inflammatory and healing, and the aroma is soothing and balancing.

## NEROLI ESSENTIAL OIL (CITRUS X AURANTIUM)

Neroli comes from the orange blossom, the flower of the bitter orange tree. Widely used to prepare cologne waters and perfumes, its aroma is intense and sweet.

It is a great cell regenerator that fights aging, hydrates the skin and reduces and prevents stretch marks. It relaxes and calms the central nervous system, and it also has aphrodisiac and energetic properties.

## YLANG YLANG ESSENTIAL OIL (CANANGA ODORATA)

A flower native to the Philippines, ylang ylang means 'flower of flowers'. Its scent is sweet and strong, reminiscent of jasmine and neroli. It's great for balancing oily skin, is anti-aging and regenerating, and also stimulates and strengthens hair.

In aromatherapy it has relaxing effects, increases joy and creativity, and has aphrodisiac properties.

## ROCK ROSE ESSENTIAL OIL (CISTUS LADANIFER)

Although the branches are used to make the essential oil, this shrub is characterised by its wonderful white and pink flowers.

It has astringent, regenerating, antiseptic and anti-inflammatory properties, and is suggested for flaccid, cracked, wrinkled, acne-prone and rosacea skin.

## CHAMOMILE ESSENTIAL OIL (CHAMAEMELUM NOBILE)

Chamomile contains many beneficial properties for our skin and our emotional state. It is extracted from the chamomile flower and has an intense and sweet aroma, like honey.

It is anti-inflammatory and healing, ideal for sensitive skin, acne-prone skin and as a hair lightener. It is calming and sedative.

## JASMINE ESSENTIAL OIL (JASMINUM OFFICINALE, JASMINUM GRANDIFLORUM)

This oil is extracted from jasmine flowers and is widely used in classic perfumery.

With a penetrating and sweet smell, it has rejuvenating effects on the skin, calms irritations and encourages elasticity. Its aphrodisiac power is well known.

## LAVENDER ESSENTIAL OIL (LAVANDULA ANGUSTIFOLIA)

This is THE essential essential oil that you should never be without. It has innumerable properties: anti-inflammatory, healing, antifungal, antiseptic, calming, sedative ...

Suitable for all skin types, you can use it in endless ways in cosmetics: for insect bites, added to a hair mask, for making deodorants, to perfume the air ...

Due to its calming and sedative scent, it is useful in stressful situations and can combat insomnia.

## ROSE ESSENTIAL OIL (ROSA X DAMASCENA)

Perhaps the queen of fragrances, the rose represents love and beauty, and its scent is delicate and sensual.

It is moisturising and anti-aging ... It calms, softens and regenerates irritated skin, and reduces scars and stretch marks. Because of its soothing smell, it's suggested for sadness, melancholy and nervous depression.

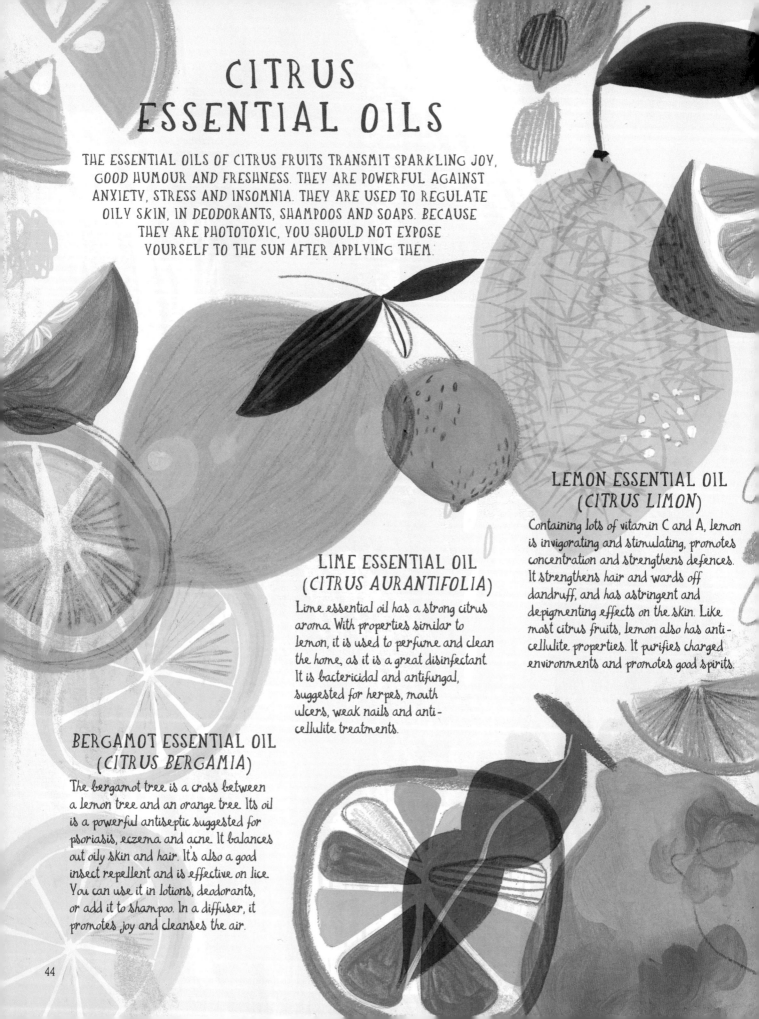

# CITRUS ESSENTIAL OILS

THE ESSENTIAL OILS OF CITRUS FRUITS TRANSMIT SPARKLING JOY, GOOD HUMOUR AND FRESHNESS. THEY ARE POWERFUL AGAINST ANXIETY, STRESS AND INSOMNIA. THEY ARE USED TO REGULATE OILY SKIN, IN DEODORANTS, SHAMPOOS AND SOAPS. BECAUSE THEY ARE PHOTOTOXIC, YOU SHOULD NOT EXPOSE YOURSELF TO THE SUN AFTER APPLYING THEM.

## LEMON ESSENTIAL OIL (CITRUS LIMON)

Containing lots of vitamin C and A, lemon is invigorating and stimulating, promotes concentration and strengthens defences. It strengthens hair and wards off dandruff, and has astringent and depigmenting effects on the skin. Like most citrus fruits, lemon also has anti-cellulite properties. It purifies charged environments and promotes good spirits.

## LIME ESSENTIAL OIL (CITRUS AURANTIFOLIA)

Lime essential oil has a strong citrus aroma. With properties similar to lemon, it is used to perfume and clean the home, as it is a great disinfectant. It is bactericidal and antifungal, suggested for herpes, mouth ulcers, weak nails and anti-cellulite treatments.

## BERGAMOT ESSENTIAL OIL (CITRUS BERGAMIA)

The bergamot tree is a cross between a lemon tree and an orange tree. Its oil is a powerful antiseptic suggested for psoriasis, eczema and acne. It balances out oily skin and hair. It's also a good insect repellent and is effective on lice. You can use it in lotions, deodorants, or add it to shampoo. In a diffuser, it promotes joy and cleanses the air.

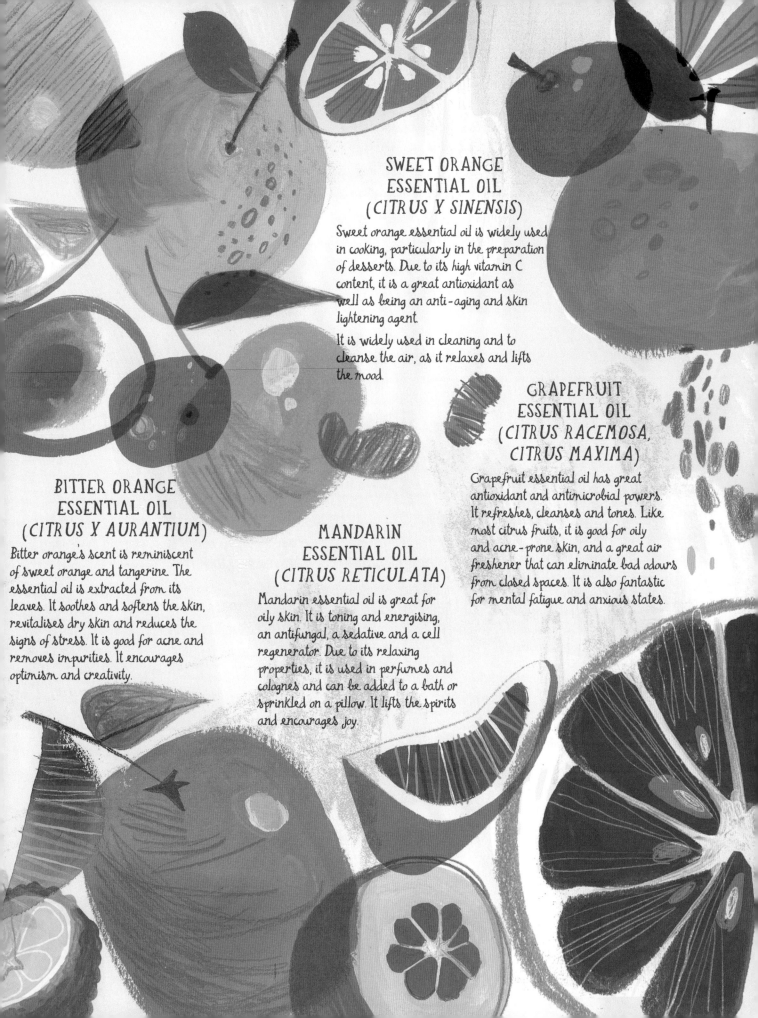

## SWEET ORANGE ESSENTIAL OIL (CITRUS X SINENSIS)

Sweet orange essential oil is widely used in cooking, particularly in the preparation of desserts. Due to its high vitamin C content, it is a great antioxidant as well as being an anti-aging and skin lightening agent.

It is widely used in cleaning and to cleanse the air, as it relaxes and lifts the mood.

## GRAPEFRUIT ESSENTIAL OIL (CITRUS RACEMOSA, CITRUS MAXIMA)

Grapefruit essential oil has great antioxidant and antimicrobial powers. It refreshes, cleanses and tones. Like most citrus fruits, it is good for oily and acne-prone skin, and a great air freshener that can eliminate bad odours from closed spaces. It is also fantastic for mental fatigue and anxious states.

## BITTER ORANGE ESSENTIAL OIL (CITRUS X AURANTIUM)

Bitter orange's scent is reminiscent of sweet orange and tangerine. The essential oil is extracted from its leaves. It soothes and softens the skin, revitalises dry skin and reduces the signs of stress. It is good for acne and removes impurities. It encourages optimism and creativity.

## MANDARIN ESSENTIAL OIL (CITRUS RETICULATA)

Mandarin essential oil is great for oily skin. It is toning and energising, an antifungal, a sedative and a cell regenerator. Due to its relaxing properties, it is used in perfumes and colognes and can be added to a bath or sprinkled on a pillow. It lifts the spirits and encourages joy.

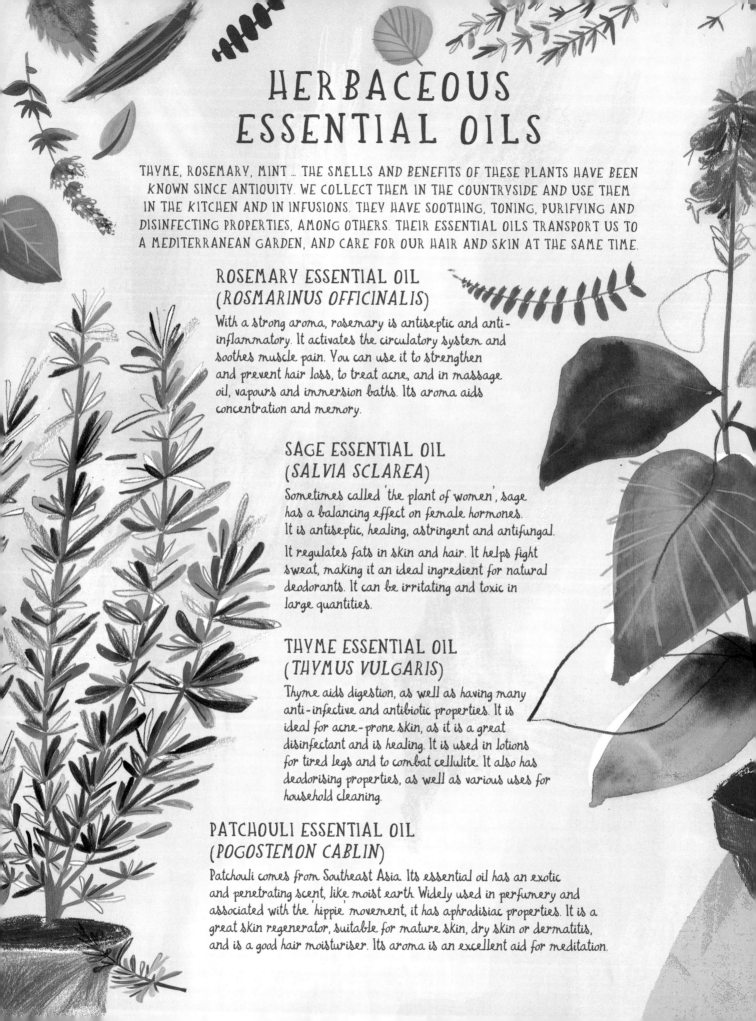

# HERBACEOUS ESSENTIAL OILS

THYME, ROSEMARY, MINT ... THE SMELLS AND BENEFITS OF THESE PLANTS HAVE BEEN KNOWN SINCE ANTIQUITY. WE COLLECT THEM IN THE COUNTRYSIDE AND USE THEM IN THE KITCHEN AND IN INFUSIONS. THEY HAVE SOOTHING, TONING, PURIFYING AND DISINFECTING PROPERTIES, AMONG OTHERS. THEIR ESSENTIAL OILS TRANSPORT US TO A MEDITERRANEAN GARDEN, AND CARE FOR OUR HAIR AND SKIN AT THE SAME TIME.

## ROSEMARY ESSENTIAL OIL
### (ROSMARINUS OFFICINALIS)

With a strong aroma, rosemary is antiseptic and anti-inflammatory. It activates the circulatory system and soothes muscle pain. You can use it to strengthen and prevent hair loss, to treat acne, and in massage oil, vapours and immersion baths. Its aroma aids concentration and memory.

## SAGE ESSENTIAL OIL
### (SALVIA SCLAREA)

Sometimes called 'the plant of women', sage has a balancing effect on female hormones. It is antiseptic, healing, astringent and antifungal.

It regulates fats in skin and hair. It helps fight sweat, making it an ideal ingredient for natural deodorants. It can be irritating and toxic in large quantities.

## THYME ESSENTIAL OIL
### (THYMUS VULGARIS)

Thyme aids digestion, as well as having many anti-infective and antibiotic properties. It is ideal for acne-prone skin, as it is a great disinfectant and is healing. It is used in lotions for tired legs and to combat cellulite. It also has deodorising properties, as well as various uses for household cleaning.

## PATCHOULI ESSENTIAL OIL
### (POGOSTEMON CABLIN)

Patchouli comes from Southeast Asia. Its essential oil has an exotic and penetrating scent, like moist earth. Widely used in perfumery and associated with the 'hippie' movement, it has aphrodisiac properties. It is a great skin regenerator, suitable for mature skin, dry skin or dermatitis, and is a good hair moisturiser. Its aroma is an excellent aid for meditation.

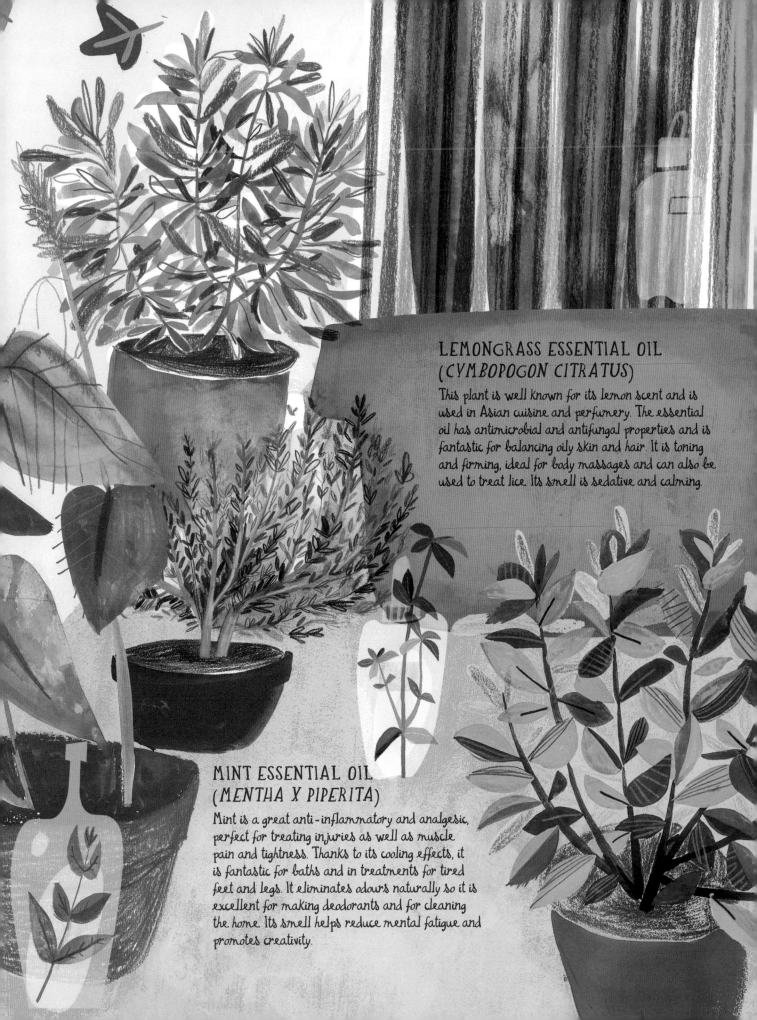

## LEMONGRASS ESSENTIAL OIL
## (CYMBOPOGON CITRATUS)

This plant is well known for its lemon scent and is used in Asian cuisine and perfumery. The essential oil has antimicrobial and antifungal properties and is fantastic for balancing oily skin and hair. It is toning and firming, ideal for body massages and can also be used to treat lice. Its smell is sedative and calming.

## MINT ESSENTIAL OIL
## (MENTHA X PIPERITA)

Mint is a great anti-inflammatory and analgesic, perfect for treating injuries as well as muscle pain and tightness. Thanks to its cooling effects, it is fantastic for baths and in treatments for tired feet and legs. It eliminates odours naturally so it is excellent for making deodorants and for cleaning the home. Its smell helps reduce mental fatigue and promotes creativity.

# TREE ESSENTIAL OILS

THE PEACE OF THE FOREST APPEARS WHEN WE INHALE ESSENTIAL OILS DERIVED FROM TREES. TAKE A WALK THROUGH THESE SCENTS AND FEEL THEIR STRENGTH AND VALUE.

MOST OF THEM STIMULATE THE IMMUNE SYSTEM AND PROTECT SKIN AGAINST EXTERNAL AGGRAVATION AND AGING.

## CYPRESS ESSENTIAL OIL (CUPRESSUS SEMPERVIRENS)

The essential oil of this Mediterranean tree is distinguished by its ability to aid decongestion and stimulate the circulatory system. It is recommended for varicose veins and tired legs, muscle pain after exercise and cellulite-reducing massages. It acts against excessive sweat.

## LAUREL ESSENTIAL OIL (LAURUS NOBILIS)

Originally from the Mediterranean, the laurel is one of the most revered trees. A common ingredient in men's cosmetics due to its spicy smell, it is a powerful antibacterial, fungicidal and analgesic. It is used in massages for muscle and joint pain, as a dandruff treatment and to strengthen the scalp. Inhaled, it promotes relaxation, concentration and memory.

## PINE ESSENTIAL OIL (PINUS SYLVESTRIS)

Suitable for respiratory conditions and muscle pain, it has a strong smell that is reminiscent of resin. It is an antiseptic, bactericide and insecticide. It relieves physical fatigue and exhaustion.
In cosmetics, it is used for massage oils, to regulate oily and acne-prone skin and as a deodorant. It's also suitable for cleaning the house.

## FRANKINCENSE ESSENTIAL OIL (BOSWELLIA SACRA)

Frankincense is the resin of an African tree that lives in very arid areas. It is a thick orange-coloured oil with a woody aroma. Associated with religious rituals and ceremonies, it aids meditative states and calmness. It is ideal to use in a diffuser while pratising yoga. In cosmetics, it prevents aging and wrinkles and has great healing powers.

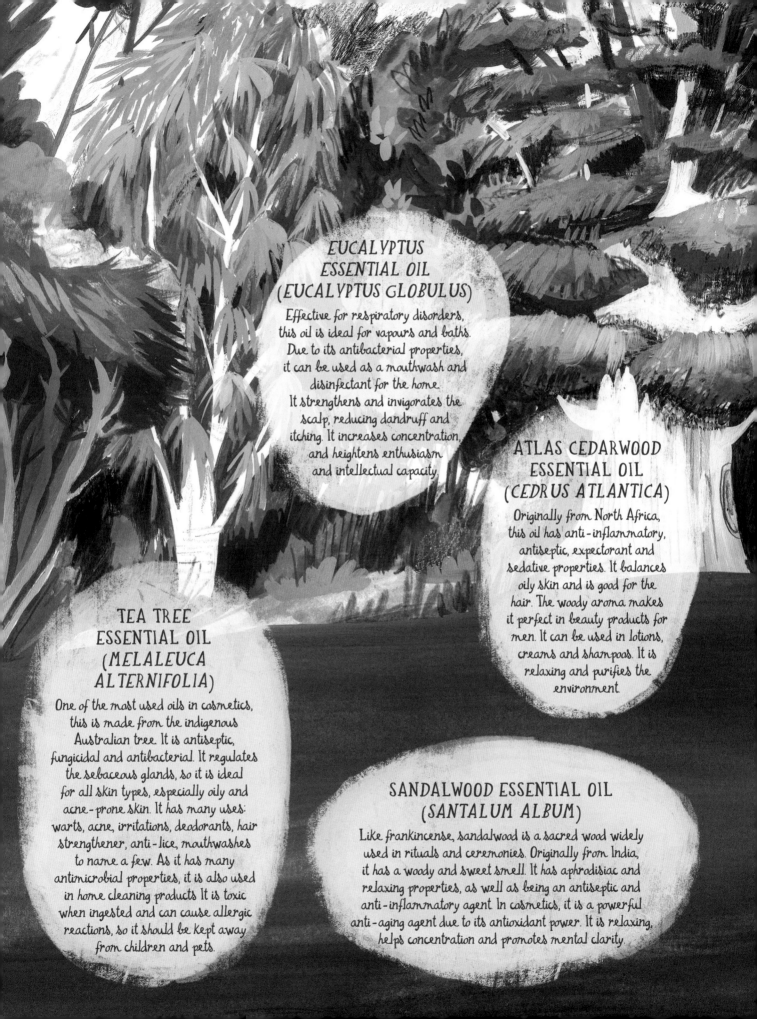

## EUCALYPTUS ESSENTIAL OIL (EUCALYPTUS GLOBULUS)

Effective for respiratory disorders, this oil is ideal for vapours and baths. Due to its antibacterial properties, it can be used as a mouthwash and disinfectant for the home. It strengthens and invigorates the scalp, reducing dandruff and itching. It increases concentration, and heightens enthusiasm and intellectual capacity.

## ATLAS CEDARWOOD ESSENTIAL OIL (CEDRUS ATLANTICA)

Originally from North Africa, this oil has anti-inflammatory, antiseptic, expectorant and sedative properties. It balances oily skin and is good for the hair. The woody aroma makes it perfect in beauty products for men. It can be used in lotions, creams and shampoos. It is relaxing and purifies the environment.

## TEA TREE ESSENTIAL OIL (MELALEUCA ALTERNIFOLIA)

One of the most used oils in cosmetics, this is made from the indigenous Australian tree. It is antiseptic, fungicidal and antibacterial. It regulates the sebaceous glands, so it is ideal for all skin types, especially oily and acne-prone skin. It has many uses: warts, acne, irritations, deodorants, hair strengthener, anti-lice, mouthwashes to name a few. As it has many antimicrobial properties, it is also used in home cleaning products. It is toxic when ingested and can cause allergic reactions, so it should be kept away from children and pets.

## SANDALWOOD ESSENTIAL OIL (SANTALUM ALBUM)

Like frankincense, sandalwood is a sacred wood widely used in rituals and ceremonies. Originally from India, it has a woody and sweet smell. It has aphrodisiac and relaxing properties, as well as being an antiseptic and anti-inflammatory agent. In cosmetics, it is a powerful anti-aging agent due to its antioxidant power. It is relaxing, helps concentration and promotes mental clarity.

# PRECAUTIONS AND USES OF ESSENTIAL OILS

EVEN THOUGH THEY ARE NATURAL PRODUCTS, ESSENTIAL OILS ARE NOT EXEMPT FROM RISKS, AS THEY ARE VERY POWERFUL CHEMICAL COMPOUNDS. USE THEM IN MODERATION AND ALWAYS WITH COMMON SENSE. THESE ARE THE PRECAUTIONS RECOMMENDED BY EXPERTS THAT YOU SHOULD CONSIDER.

- Do not use orally without medical supervision. Although some forms of aromatherapy use them internally, they should not be ingested without specialised medical supervision. In the event of accidental ingestion, you must seek medical treatment or go to a hospital.

- They should NOT be used by pregnant people, children or the elderly. Although some oils are very mild, you should still consult a specialist if you are planning to use them. If you have any type of disease or neurological condition, you should also consult a specialist.

- Never apply them directly to the skin. Always dilute them with a vegetable carrier oil.

- Avoid contact with the eyes and mucus membranes, as the oils can be irritating. In the event of contact with these areas, apply a vegetable oil, rinse with plenty of water and seek medical treatment if needed. Wash your hands after handling essential oils.

- Citrus essential oils are photosensitive, which can cause unwanted reactions if your skin is exposed to the sun after applying them. Use them in winter months or overnight. Keep them in the fridge once opened.

- If you have allergies, do a tolerance or patch test by applying a couple of drops in the crease of your elbow and waiting to see if there is a reaction.

- Follow the recommended dosage. Essential oils should not exceed 1.5% of the total volume in a facial preparations, and 2.5% in body preparations.

- Make sure essential oils are chemotyped*, that their origin and composition are detailed on the packaging and that they are certified by a laboratory that offers guarantees of purity and safety.

\* The chemotype of an essential oil is the most abundant aromatic molecule in it and, therefore, the one that defines it. For example, in the case of the rosemary essential oil, we found three essential oils: rosemary with camphor chemotype, rosemary with cineole chemotype and rosemary with verbenone chemotype. Although botanically they are all from the same species, because the plants are grown in different geographical environments, soils, levels of insulation, etc., individual plants have different characteristics in their essential oil and, therefore, different properties.

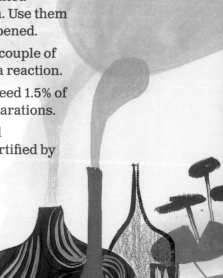

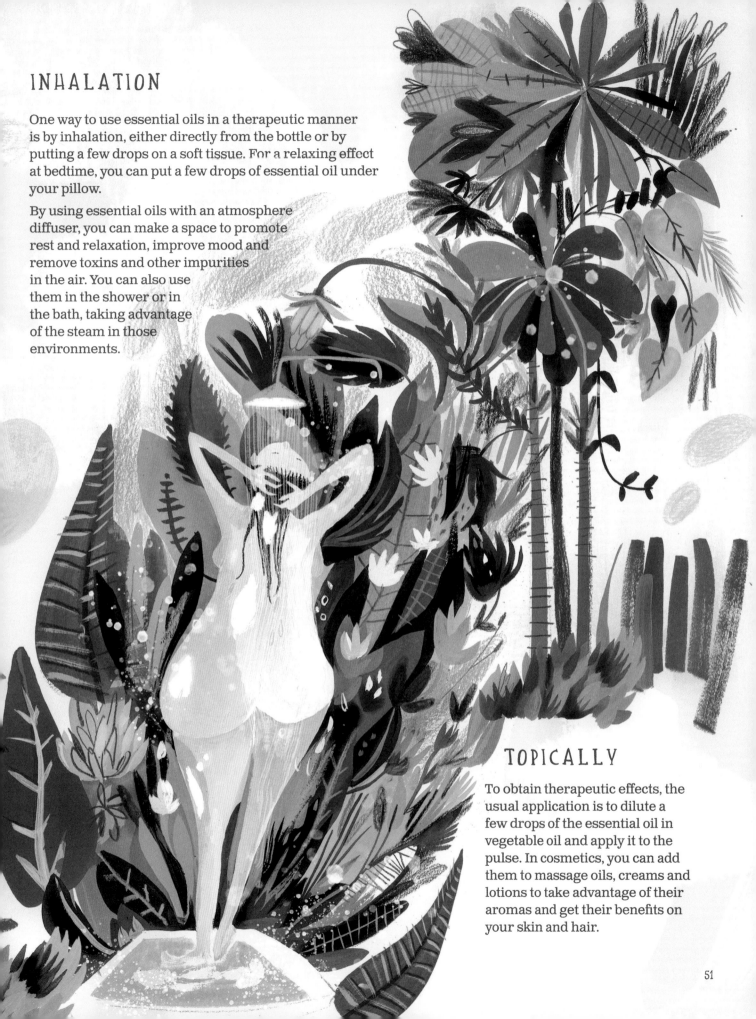

# INHALATION

One way to use essential oils in a therapeutic manner is by inhalation, either directly from the bottle or by putting a few drops on a soft tissue. For a relaxing effect at bedtime, you can put a few drops of essential oil under your pillow.

By using essential oils with an atmosphere diffuser, you can make a space to promote rest and relaxation, improve mood and remove toxins and other impurities in the air. You can also use them in the shower or in the bath, taking advantage of the steam in those environments.

# TOPICALLY

To obtain therapeutic effects, the usual application is to dilute a few drops of the essential oil in vegetable oil and apply it to the pulse. In cosmetics, you can add them to massage oils, creams and lotions to take advantage of their aromas and get their benefits on your skin and hair.

51

# ESSENTIAL OILS AND EMOTIONS

SMELLS ARE CONNECTED TO OUR MEMORIES AND OUR EMOTIONS. WHETHER USED IN A BATH, A MASSAGE OIL, A DIFFUSER OR A COUPLE OF DROPS ON A TISSUE, SCENTS CAN HELP US FEEL BETTER. CLOSE YOUR EYES, TAKE A DEEP BREATH AND ENJOY A CONNECTION WITH NATURE WHEREVER YOU ARE. HERE ARE SOME SUGGESTIONS TO HELP YOU FOSTER DIFFERENT STATES*

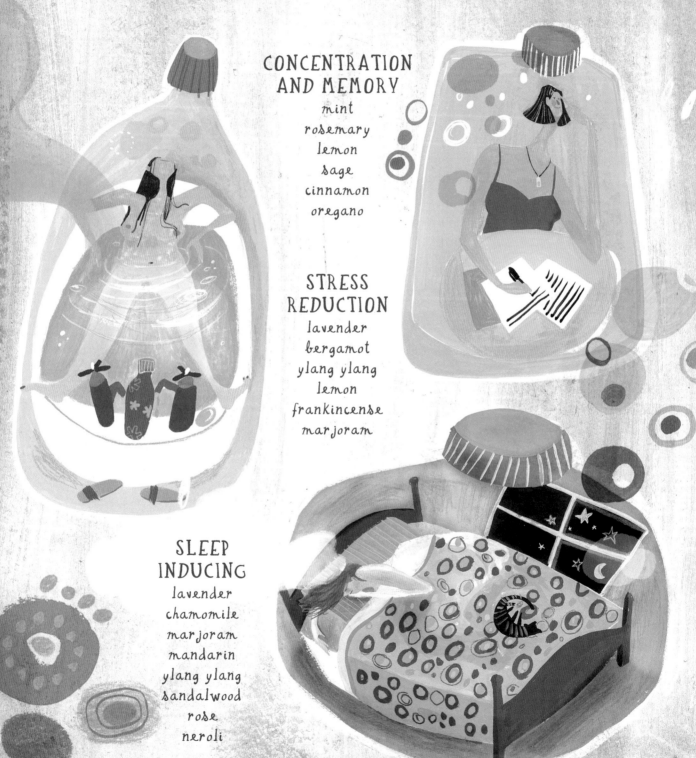

### CONCENTRATION AND MEMORY
mint
rosemary
lemon
sage
cinnamon
oregano

### STRESS REDUCTION
lavender
bergamot
ylang ylang
lemon
frankincense
marjoram

### SLEEP INDUCING
lavender
chamomile
marjoram
mandarin
ylang ylang
sandalwood
rose
neroli

* Remember to follow the precautions for use (page 50) and that essential oils must not be used by pregnant, breastfeeding or elderly people, or if you have any disease or medical condition. Always consult your doctor or your therapist.

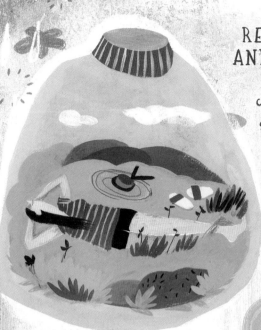

## RELAXING/ ANXIOLYTICS

lavender
chamomile
geranium
angelica
neroli
rose
pine

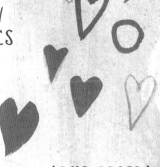

## APHRODISIAC

ylang ylang
cinnamon
ginger
sandalwood
jasmine
rose

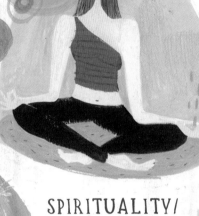

## STIMULANTS/ ENERGISERS

rosemary
grapefruit
mint
basil
cypress

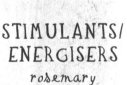

## SPIRITUALITY/ MEDITATION

frankincense
myrrh
cedar
sandalwood
neroli
patchouli
rose

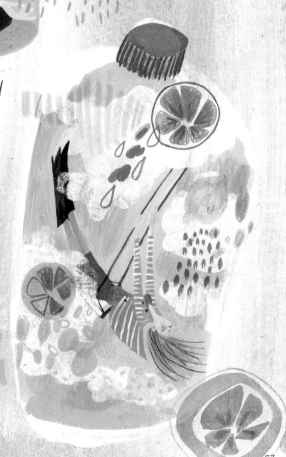

## HAPPINESS

bergamot
mandarin
basil
rosemary
ylang ylang
geranium

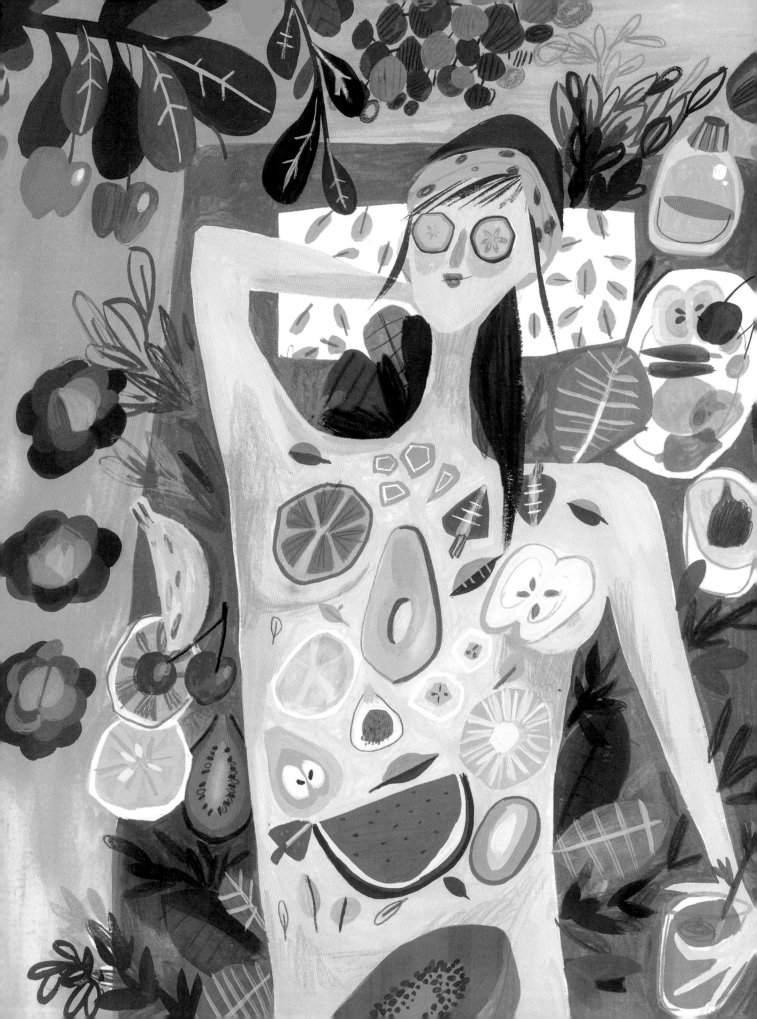

# Fruits, vegetables and fresh produce

We have incorporated purifying diets and green juices into our eating habits, and we know perfectly well all the healthy properties that vegetables, fruits and fresh produce offer our bodies. However, we tend to only use them on our skin when they are depicted on a package, and we often don't worry about how much real fruit is actually inside.

If nature is popular in cosmetics, then what could be more natural than getting it directly from the source?

If you already buy fresh, organically grown produce to eat, you can keep a small portion to treat your body. You can make fresh masks, scrubs or toners that cleanse, nourish, soothe, tone or hydrate your skin, are easy to prepare and are not expensive.

Fresh produce has concentrated amounts of many properties and active ingredients, but remember that they do not last long. In most cases, they must be prepared and used immediately, just like a salad or juice.

I suggest that, when you use fresh produce in your diet, you take advantage of it and cook for your skin too.

Can you imagine a spa in the middle of an orchard?

# FROM THE GARDEN TO YOUR SKIN: FRUITS AND VEGETABLES

APPLE, CHERRY, BANANA ... THEY ARE OFTEN GUEST STARS IN TRENDY COSMETICS. MOST OF THE BENEFITS COME FROM THEIR ANTIOXIDANT PROPERTIES AND VITAMIN CONTENT.

## BANANA
This fruit is high in minerals and vitamins. Its antioxidant, anti-inflammatory and moisturising properties stand out. Recommended for oily and acne-prone skin, it also moisturises and nourishes the hair. Banana peel is fantastic for reducing bags under eyes, soothing insect bites and even moisturising the skin.

## GRAPES
Crushed whole grapes, including the seeds, are a powerful exfoliant and antioxidant due to their polyphenol content, which tones and cleanses the skin.

## KIWI
Due to its high concentration of vitamin C, kiwi is a powerful antioxidant and regulator for oily skin. It fights cell aging and brightens the skin. Widely used in hair masks.

## MANGO
With a high beta-carotene content, mango hydrates and cleanses the dermis, purifies oily skin and is excellent for preventing hair loss.

## PAPAYA
Papaya is a great exfoliant that removes dead skin cells, brightens and moisturises.

## CITRUS FRUITS
Citrus fruits are high in vitamin C.

Lemon is astringent and exfoliating. It brightens the skin, strengthens nails and hair and is ideal for combating blackheads and pimples (but please stay out of the sun after using it).

Orange contains beta-carotene, folic acid, potassium and magnesium, and is notable for its great anti-aging power and anti-wrinkle properties.

## APPLE
Apple has antioxidant, exfoliating, toning and antiseptic properties. Fantastic for acne and sunburn relief.

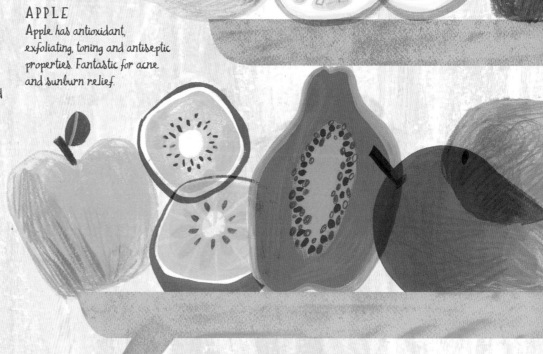

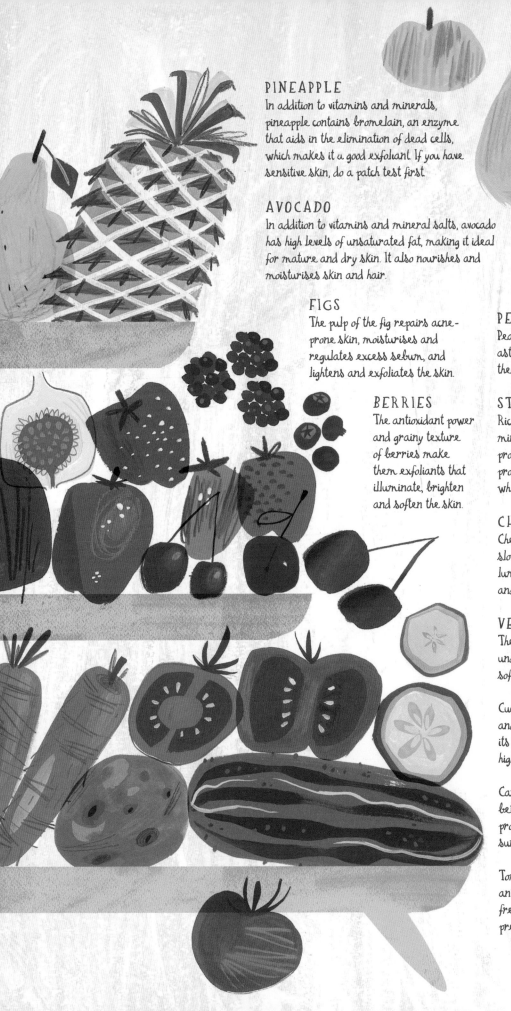

## PINEAPPLE

In addition to vitamins and minerals, pineapple contains bromelain, an enzyme that aids in the elimination of dead cells, which makes it a good exfoliant. If you have sensitive skin, do a patch test first.

## AVOCADO

In addition to vitamins and mineral salts, avocado has high levels of unsaturated fat, making it ideal for mature and dry skin. It also nourishes and moisturises skin and hair.

## FIGS

The pulp of the fig repairs acne-prone skin, moisturises and regulates excess sebum, and lightens and exfoliates the skin.

## BERRIES

The antioxidant power and grainy texture of berries make them exfoliants that illuminate, brighten and soften the skin.

## PEAR

Pears are a powerful antioxidant and astringent that cleanse, tone and purify the skin. Ideal for oily skin.

## STRAWBERRIES

Rich in vitamin A, C, folate and minerals, strawberries have astringent properties and regulate oily and acne-prone skin. They fight wrinkles and, when crushed, are a fantastic exfoliant.

## CHERRIES

Cherries are great antioxidants that slow down cellular aging and provide luminosity. They are anti-inflammatory and brighten the skin.

## VEGETABLES

The potato is known to reduce bags under the eyes as well, to brighten and soften the skin.

Cucumber purifies, refreshes, hydrates and calms the skin. In a mask or juice, its toning and cleansing properties are highly effective for the face.

Carrot is loaded with vitamins and beta-carotene, which stimulate collagen production, lengthen your tan and repair sun damage.

Tomato contains lycopene, a powerful antioxidant that protects cells from free radicals. It is also exfoliating and prevents blemishes.

# COSMETICS FROM YOUR KITCHEN

DID YOU KNOW THAT YOUR PANTRY AND FRIDGE CONTAIN INGREDIENTS THAT YOU CAN INCORPORATE INTO YOUR DAILY BEAUTY ROUTINE? THEY MAY NOT SEEM GLAMOROUS, BUT MANY OF THEM HAVE INCREDIBLE PROPERTIES TO HELP YOUR SKIN AND HAIR. HONEY, EGGS, OATS, SALT - ALL CAN BECOME THE MAIN INGREDIENTS OF A FANTASTIC BEAUTY REGIME.

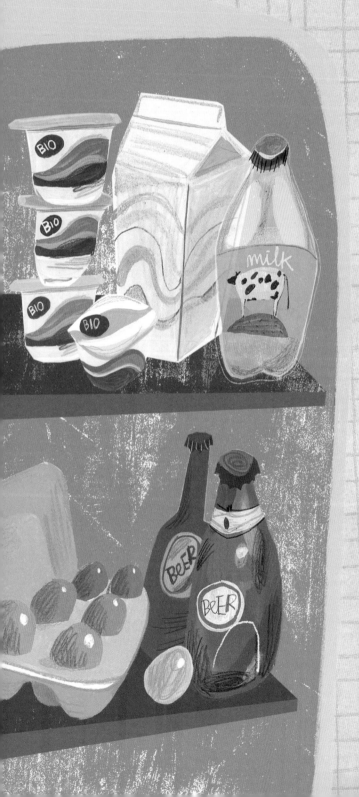

## DAIRY PRODUCTS

The lactic acid in milk and its derivatives has lots of cosmetic properties. Bioproteins retain moisture in the skin and biotin protects against external irritations. Milk is moisturising, exfoliating, regenerating and brightens the skin. Combined with oatmeal and honey, it makes a powerful treatment mask.

Yoghurt has many of the same properties, and also, due to its acidic nature and zinc content, it fights acne and exfoliates deeply. Its texture makes it perfect for masks, and it can be combined with fruit, egg or honey. It also moisturises and repairs hair.

## BEER

Beer balances acidity, softens and gives shine to hair, as well as lightening blonde hair. Yeast and hops contain B vitamins and silicon that hydrate and prevent aging.

Brewer's yeast is also fantastic for making purifying masks for acne-prone skin.

## EGGS

Egg yolk has concentrated fatty acids, proteins and cholesterol, which are great for nourishing and moisturising the hair and face. Ideal for dry and damaged skin.

Egg white has moisturising and purifying properties. It produces a lifting effect in facial masks and is great for fighting acne.

## TEA

All varieties of tea have beneficial properties, but the most outstanding are their antioxidant powers. Tea protects against aging, is a decongestant, illuminates the skin, tones and cleanses the pores, and reduces the appearance of dark circles.

## SPICES AND SEEDS

Turmeric is anti-inflammatory, regulates facial fat and brightens. Cinnamon is an ideal antiseptic, has microbial properties for acne and softens hands and feet. Ginger is an antioxidant and antibacterial and activates circulation.

## SALT, SUGAR AND VINEGAR

Salt and sugar are wonderful exfoliators - salt for the body and rough areas and sugar for the face and sensitive areas. Salt is also fantastic for relaxing baths.

Apple cider vinegar is a good regulating and anti-dandruff tonic for hair. It relaxes and reduces inflammation of the feet and body.

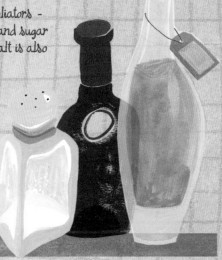

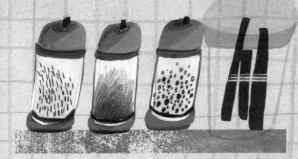

## HONEY

Its properties are innumerable: antioxidising, nourishing, antibacterial, moisturising, anti-inflammatory ... Applied alone or mixed with yoghurt, banana or oatmeal, it is a real beauty treat. Regenerates and nourishes mature skin and soothes sensitive skin. Conditions and moisturises the hair.

## RICE

Already used in cosmetics by Japanese and Korean cultures. You can use it crushed as a scrub, or boiled as an astringent and lightening mask.

In water, it is a wonderful facial toner, ideal for refining pores.

## OATS

Oats have a softening, calming and relaxing effect on dry and inflamed skin. Oatmeal creates a thin layer that prevents skin dehydration. Fantastic as a scrub, toner and in baths and soaps.

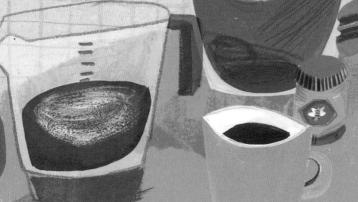

## COFFEE AND COCOA

Because of its caffeine content, coffee fights cellulite (coffee grounds make a wonderful exfoliant). It strengthens and activates the scalp, and invigorates the eye contour.

Cocoa fights aging due to its antioxidant properties. It is exfoliating, anti-inflammatory and improves circulation. Masks and scrubs made with cocoa are a pleasure for all the senses.

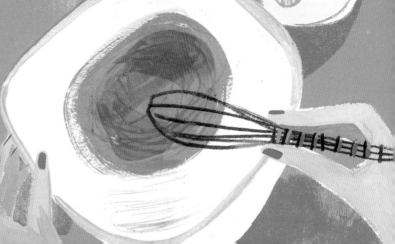

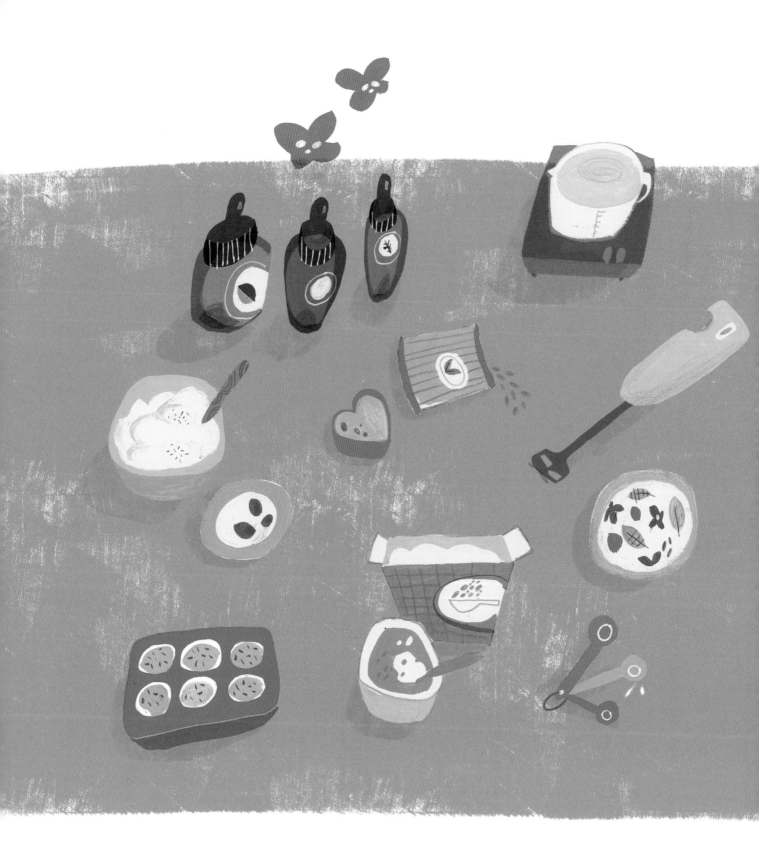

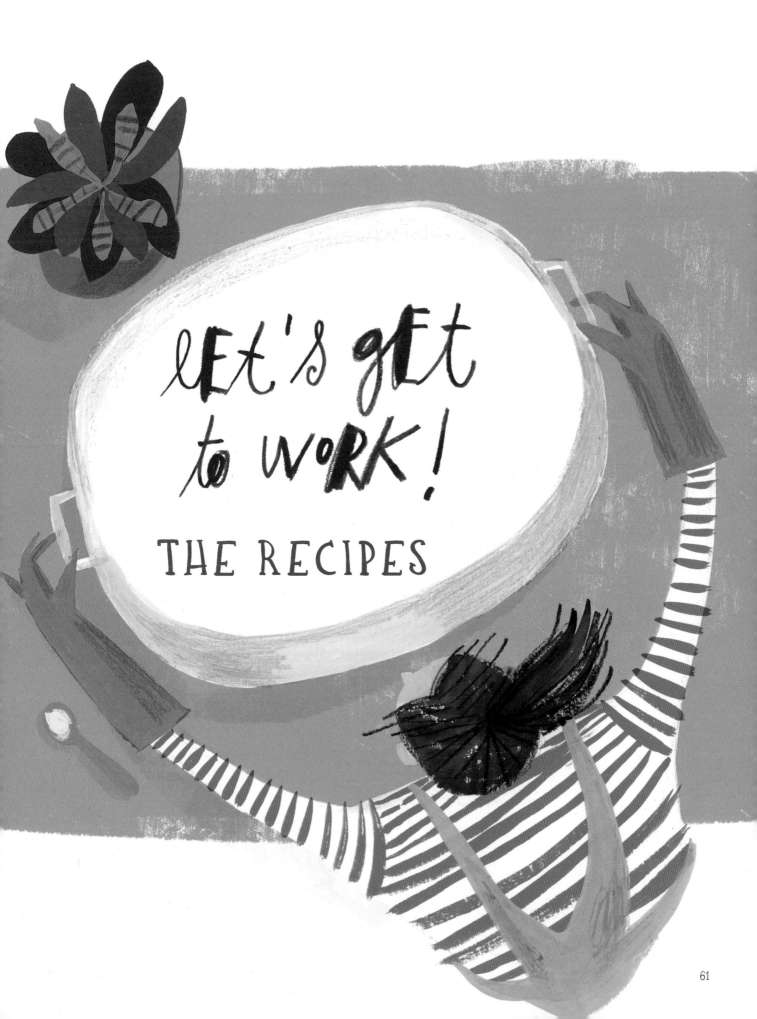

let's get to work!

THE RECIPES

# BEFORE STARTING

The long-awaited moment has arrived, but before you begin, read these tips and guidelines so that everything goes according to plan.

- Switching to natural cosmetics is not a huge change. You don't have to throw away all your products at once and start fervently making creams and potions. And you don't have to buy everything. I suggest you start with the simplest recipes, like fruit masks, oil serums or scrubs, and introduce new ingredients, little by little, and in small quantities.

- I'm not saying that you stop buying conventional cosmetics or stop going to your beautician or hairdresser. Whatever you do will be perfect, because what matters most is that you are free to choose what you want.

- Essential oils and ingredients for making cosmetics are popular and widely available, but check the quality and origin of products sold online. The ingredients you use must be natural or organically produced.

- Precisely because they are of natural origin, some foods or essential oils can cause allergies or skin irritations. If you have any type of food intolerance or reactive skin, always do a patch test in the elbow crease to check for any reaction.

- Natural cosmetics expire quickly, especially those that contain water. There are certified ecological preservatives that will extend the life of your creams by around 3 months (at most, depending on the season and the method of conservation). Make small batches and store them in the fridge. If you notice any changes in colour, odour or texture, play it safe and throw it away.

- The texture and absorption time of some creams or oils are not the same as conventional products, and their consistency can change depending on the time of year.

- The area where you are going to make your cosmetics, and the equipment you are going to use, must be clean and well disinfected. Sterilise and clean all utensils with alcohol. This equipment should be reserved exclusively for making your cosmetics.

- You must be very scrupulous with hygiene to keep the environment clean. Wash your hands well and wear gloves if you can. All these precautions will extend the life of your products.

- Keep the ingredients in a dark and dry place so they don't spoil.

- Store natural cosmetics in sterilised glass jars. Try to recycle as much as you can.

- Label your natural cosmetics with the date and formula (or create a reference so you can locate this information). I recommend that you start a notebook to record your formulas, dates, drawings of the process and observations of each cosmetic once you have made it.

- Design cute labels and give your creations fun names.

- Measurements have been given as cups, spoons, drops, grams and millimetres. Don't be put off if you usually measure things in imperial units (i.e. ounces and fluid ounces). Use your precision weighing scales set to the 'gram' setting to measure as required.

# GUIDANCE TABLES

Although the proportions are always indicative, below are some measurements that will help when making your cosmetics.

1 small cup
= 150 ml (5 fl oz)

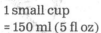

1 tablespoon
= 15 ml (½ fl oz)

1 teaspoon
= 5 ml (¼ fl oz)

weight of
1 tablespoon

water = 15 g (½ oz)

approximate dosages for essential oil (for 50 ml/1¾ fl oz):
diffusers: 5 to 10 drops

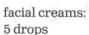

facial creams:
5 drops

massage oil or cream: 12 drops

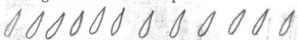

1 ml of essential oil = 20 drops

oil = 15 g (½ oz)

sugar = 12.5 g (⅓ oz)

flour = 8 g (¼ oz)

standard volumes
of packaging

  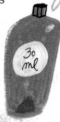 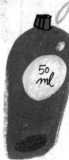 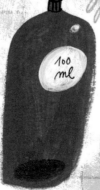

5 ml   10 ml   30 ml   50 ml   100 ml

cornflour
(cornstarch) =
12 g (⅓ oz)

63

# UTENSILS

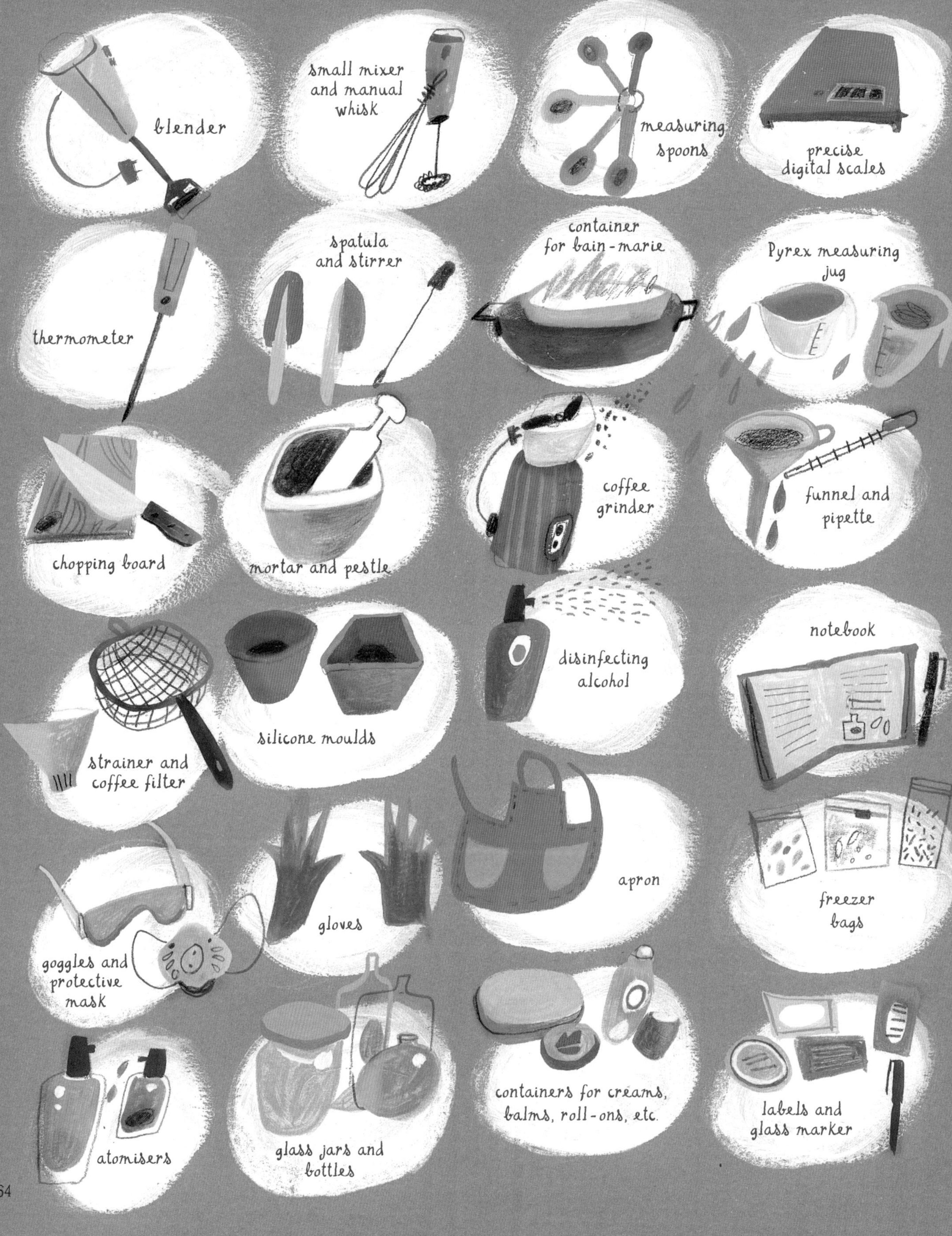

blender

small mixer and manual whisk

measuring spoons

precise digital scales

thermometer

spatula and stirrer

container for bain-marie

Pyrex measuring jug

chopping board

mortar and pestle

coffee grinder

funnel and pipette

strainer and coffee filter

silicone moulds

disinfecting alcohol

notebook

goggles and protective mask

gloves

apron

freezer bags

atomisers

glass jars and bottles

containers for creams, balms, roll-ons, etc.

labels and glass marker

# RAW MATERIALS

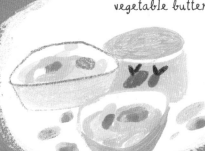

vegetable butters

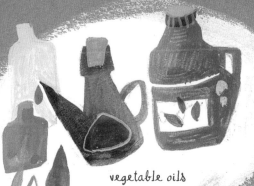

vegetable oils

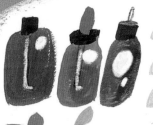

essential oils

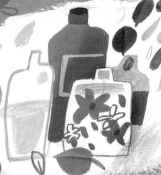

hydrosols or floral waters

flowers and medicinal plants

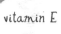

vitamin E

natural additives (honey, vinegar, oatmeal, salt, clay, etc.)

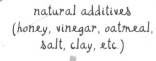

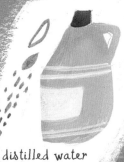

distilled water

authorised preservatives

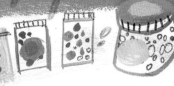

emulsifying waxes

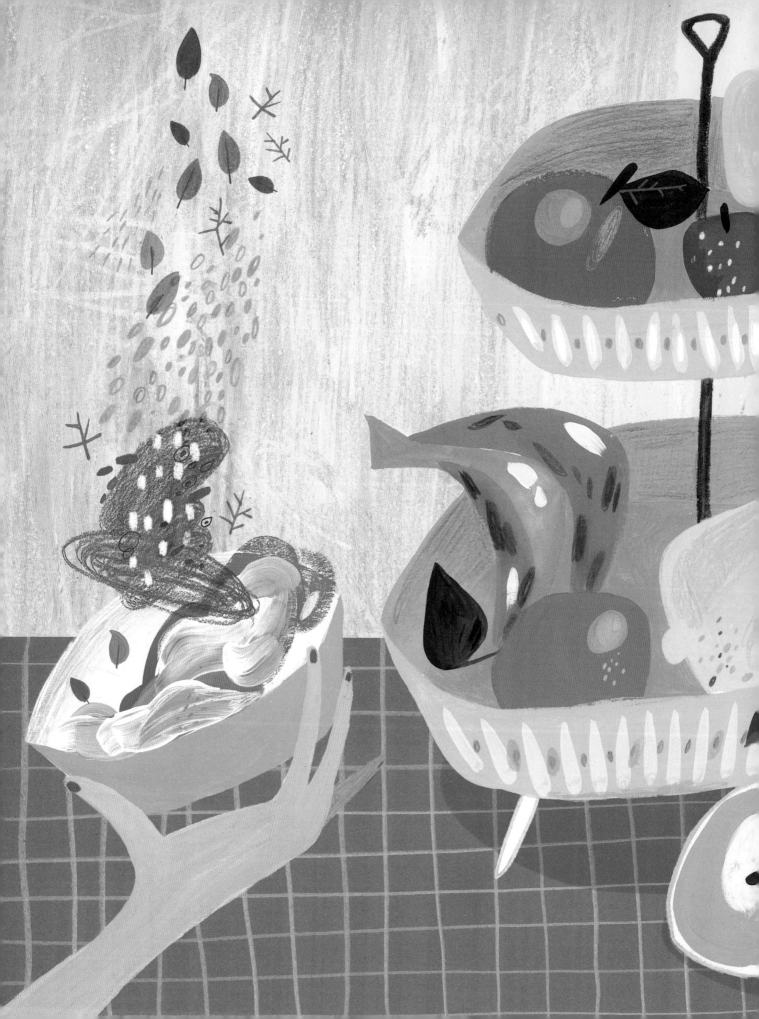

# fACE mASKs

A simple banana or a lone, sad yoghurt abandoned in a corner of the fridge can be fantastic allies for your skin. We are so used to needing things to be glamorous (fabulous packaging, important-sounding technical names, miraculous properties, etc.) that we end up buying products that have fruit pictured on the label ... But don't you think it might be better to use the real fruit?

It seems that fruits and fresh produce lose their value when pitted against coloured boxes and slick marketing campaigns. Freshness only has one price, and that is time, as fresh products expire quickly. I encourage you to be open to cross over in your beauty routines – keep in mind that your kitchen and your fridge are full of products that can take very good care of your skin.

If you want to convert to natural skin care, you must change your way of thinking, learn what products are good for you and use them accordingly. The same can be said for essential oils, vegetable oils and clays. They are raw materials that you must acknowledge as authentic and real cosmetics that only need a little of your handiwork and love to become effective treatments.

Fresh fruits, cereals, flours, oils, vegetables, dairy products, eggs and honey can all benefit your skin. Most fresh produce has beneficial components, such as lactic acid, glycolic acid, antioxidants, vitamin C, beta-carotene, fatty acids ... You just need to familiarise yourself with them and learn to combine them.

Other great products, such as clay or activated carbon, have endless expiration dates and are prepared by mixing with water. I beg you not to stop trying them.

Do you spend time meditating, watching a TV series, listening to a podcast or on social media? You can do all that while wearing a mask. It takes just 15 minutes.

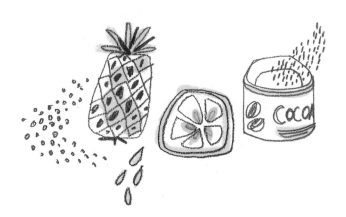

# FIFTEEN MINUTES OF LOVE

Almost all fruits and vegetables have beneficial properties. The dream is to find that perfect combination that suits your needs. Treat yourself to a wonderful, easy and inexpensive treatment. It only takes 15 minutes.

## NUTRITION AND REGENERATION: AVOCADO, BANANA AND HONEY

Using a fork, mash a banana and half an avocado together. Stir in a tablespoon of honey. Apply it to your face and let it work for 15 minutes. Remove the mask with lukewarm water then hydrate with a rose hydrosol.

## TONING, MOISTURISING AND SOOTHING: CUCUMBER, YOGHURT AND ALOE

This super-refreshing mask is the ideal treatment after a day at the beach, during hot weather or to clear your head in the morning. Take a cucumber, reserving a couple of beautiful slices for your eyes (pop them in the freezer for now). Puree the rest, add 60 g (1/4 cup) yoghurt, and a drop of mint essential oil (optional). Apply it to your face and place the cold cucumber slices on your eyes. Leave for 10 to 15 minutes, then remove it with a homemade tonic made of fresh water and a teaspoon of vinegar.

## DECONGESTANT AND BRIGHTENING: THE POTATO

Bags under your eyes? Puffy face? Stains? A simple potato can do a lot. Take a potato, wash it a little and peel it. Place some of the skins in the freezer while you prepare the rest. Grate or mash the potato and add 1 tablespoon of powdered milk or 2 tablespoons of yoghurt. Spread the mixture over your face, then take the skins out of the freezer and put them around your eyes (eyelids and bags) for 15 minutes. Remove the mask with a hydrosol.

## TWO-IN-ONE: NOURISHING EGG-BASED MASK FOR FACE AND HAIR

Take an egg and separate the yolk and white. In a bowl, mix the yolk with 2 tablespoons of olive oil and 1 tablespoon of brewer's yeast. Mix well and apply it to the hair, in particular from mid-length to the ends of damaged hair. Wrap in a towel and leave to work. Beat the egg white and apply it to the eyelid and eye contour area using a cotton pad. To the rest of the egg white, add a tablespoon of honey and a splash of almond or olive oil. Spread it over the rest of the face and neck. Rest for 10 minutes then remove the masks under the shower.

## A PERFECT BREAKFAST INSIDE AND OUT: OATMEAL, HONEY AND YOGHURT

Mix a couple of tablespoons of oatmeal with 60 g (1/4 cup) yoghurt, then leave for a few minutes, which allows the oatmeal to soften. Add 1 tablespoon of honey and mix well. Apply it to the face and leave it for 15 minutes, then rinse with water.

## MATCHA TEA: ANTIOXIDANTS AND MINERALS

Enjoy the cosmetic properties of matcha tea, loaded with antioxidants that will help delay your skin aging.

Oily skin: 2 tablespoons of aloe vera, 1 tablespoon of matcha tea, 1 teaspoon of cornflour (cornstarch) and 1 drop of tea tree essential oil. Mix it up and apply to your face. Wait about 10 minutes then rinse with warm water.

Dry skin: mix 2 tablespoons of yoghurt, 1 tablespoon of matcha tea, 1 tablespoon of honey and 1 teaspoon of almond oil in a bowl, then apply. Wait 10 to 15 minutes then rinse with water.

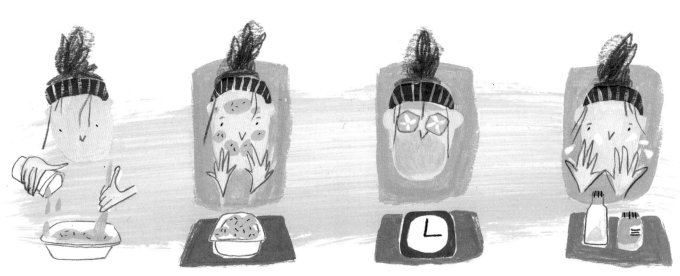

# DEAR CLAYS

Clays are the product of rock erosion caused by wind, sea and rain. They are mineral substances used since time immemorial for multiple purposes. Their healing power and cosmetic properties should not be underestimated. When mixed with water, they turn into a paste that can be applied as a mask on a specific area of the skin. They regulate fat, cleanse, soothe, hydrate, purify ... Their properties are incredible.

Clays have a fantastic consistency that allows you to add vegetable oils and essential oils to make great beauty treatments. They concentrate the power and strength of the earth so we can use them on our skin. I love them.

## KAOLIN (WHITE CLAY)

Recommended for normal, dry and sensitive skin, and ideal for dermatitis, this clay cleanses the pores without removing all the oil from the skin, maintaining its level of hydration. Provides a tightening effect that can be seen immediately. Soothes skin irritations caused by changes in the weather or too much sun. The lesser-known yellow clay has similar properties.

## BASE RECIPE

Place 2 tablespoons of clay in a bowl. Add warm water, little by little, mixing, to form a paste. You can replace the water with a hydrosol (see page 101) or infusion, and add some vegetable oil, essential oil, yoghurt, honey, etc. I prepare them in a small bowl and mix them with a spatula. Apply it with a brush or your fingers and, before it is completely dry, remove it with warm water.

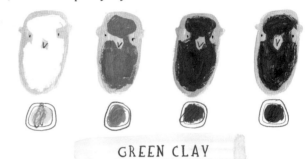

## GREEN CLAY

Used for oily and acne-prone skin, it is a strong astringent with detoxifying powers and high bactericidal properties. Deeply cleanses and purifies the skin. Only apply it in the T-zone of combination skin.

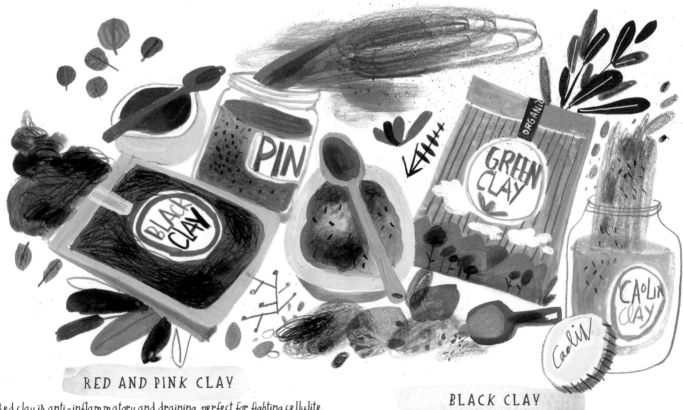

## RED AND PINK CLAY

Red clay is anti-inflammatory and draining, perfect for fighting cellulite and for body treatments. It is revitalising and energising, ideal for muscle pain. Regenerates collagen and elastin in the skin. Pink clay is made from a mixture of red and white clay, offering the properties of both clays.

## BLACK CLAY

Very fashionable! The black colour is due to its high manganese content. With a high purifying and astringent power, it is credited with the ability to counteract skin problems caused by pollution. Healing and regenerating.

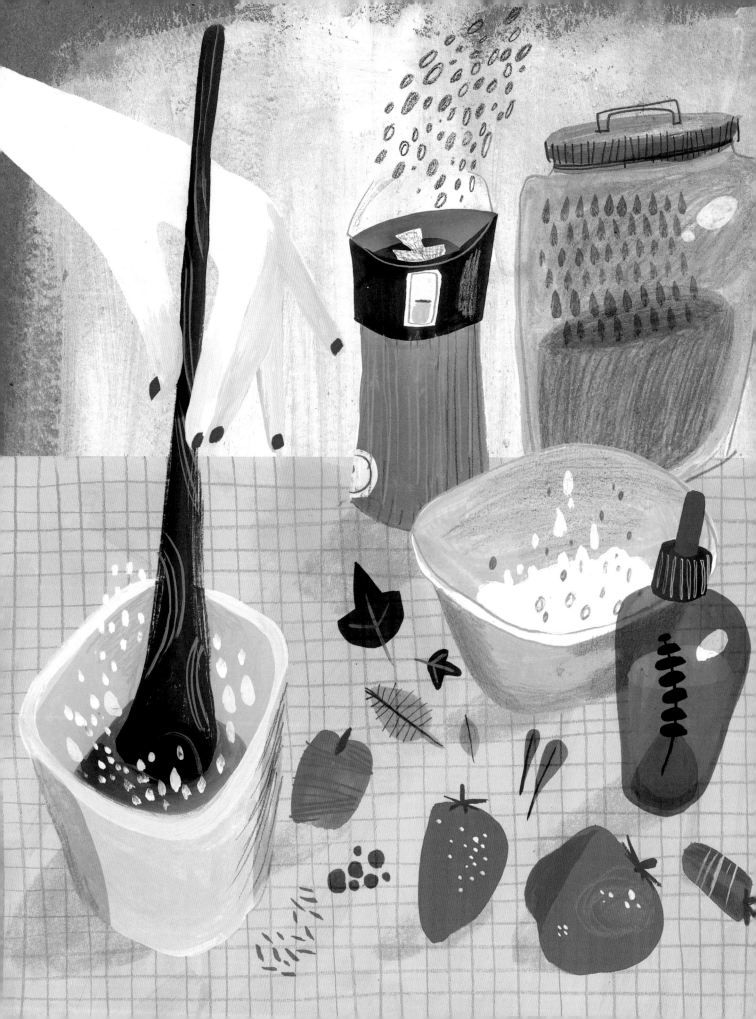

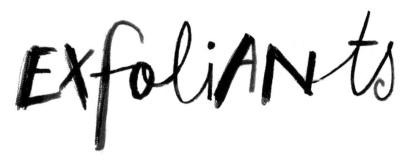

# EXfoliANts

Our skin is always in a process of cell renewal. Exfoliating helps to speed up this process by removing dead cells that accumulate on the epidermis. After exfoliating, your skin will look healthier, breathe better and absorb treatments more effectively.

There are many natural products that you can use to exfoliate the skin. They work either mechanically, using friction, or chemically, using the acids contained in some fresh produce, fresh fruit and dairy products.

The usual recommendation is to exfoliate once a week for normal skin, once every fortnight for sensitive skin and twice a week for mature skin. It is not recommended that you exfoliate excessively, because the effect could be counterproductive: you can damage the lipid layer that protects your skin. Use fine textures on the face and a coarser grain for the body, concentrating on knees, elbows and heels.

Always exfoliate on damp skin then hydrate it well. Ideally, exfoliate at night before going to bed. If you do it in the morning, it is important to use sun protection afterwards if you are going to expose your skin to the sun.

There are many basic exfoliating products that you can find in your kitchen: sugar, salt, honey, oatmeal, almonds, rice, coffee, baking soda, yoghurt and milk, as well as fruits such as strawberries, apple, kiwi and lemon to which you can add crushed dry flowers, clays and essential oils. Always add vegetable oil to emulsify the mixture and incorporate moisturising properties into your homemade scrub.

Dry brushing, based on the Garshana Ayurvedic ritual, is done with a brush containing soft natural bristles. Use the brush to rub your body with gentle movements towards the heart, respecting the delicate areas. This ritual is performed in the morning, before entering the shower. In addition to exfoliating, it activates circulation (perfect for cellulite!) and will give you vitality and energy to face a long day.

Horsehair mittens and loofah sponges for the body are also good mechanical exfoliators, but should always be used wet. For the face, you can use a konjac sponge, which comes from Korea. If you use these types of products, keep in mind that being in a humid environment can encourage the accumulation of micro-organisms and bacteria. Store them in spaces where they can dry well after use, and wash them (with vinegar or baking soda) periodically.

There are DIY crafting techniques to make mittens and exfoliating crochet discs, which can be woven with natural cotton fibres or hemp, for example. Make sure they are soft on your skin and can be easily washed.

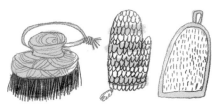

# FACIAL SCRUBS

Exfoliation is a wonderful beauty ritual, but perform it wisely. Do not exceed two exfoliations per week. Remember to always moisturise your skin afterwards and use sun protection if you are going to go outside. If you have reactive, acne-prone or sensitive skin, do not use aggressive or coarse-grained exfoliants. Instead, try Kaolin (white clay), almond flour or rice.

### EXPRESS FACIAL SCRUB

When you are short on time and need to brighten your skin, I recommend caster (superfine) sugar or panela sugar and olive oil. Sugar is already an exfoliating substance as it contains glycolic acid, in addition to the physical exfoliating effect of the granules. However, avoid it if you have sensitive skin or are going out in the sun.

In a bowl, mix 2 tablespoons of caster (superfine) sugar or panela sugar and add olive oil to create a homogeneous paste. Apply the mixture to your damp face, using gentle circular movements (without squeezing!), avoiding the skin around the eyes. Take the opportunity to also gently exfoliate the lips. Remove the scrub with warm water and dry well. Don't forget to hydrate afterwards.

### EXFOLIATING OAT MASK

There are many studies that prove the benefits of oatmeal for skin health. This oatmeal-based scrub is suitable for most skin types. It is moisturising, soothing, anti-inflammatory and cleansing. Enrich it and give it a wonderful texture with the addition of honey and yoghurt.

In a bowl, mix:

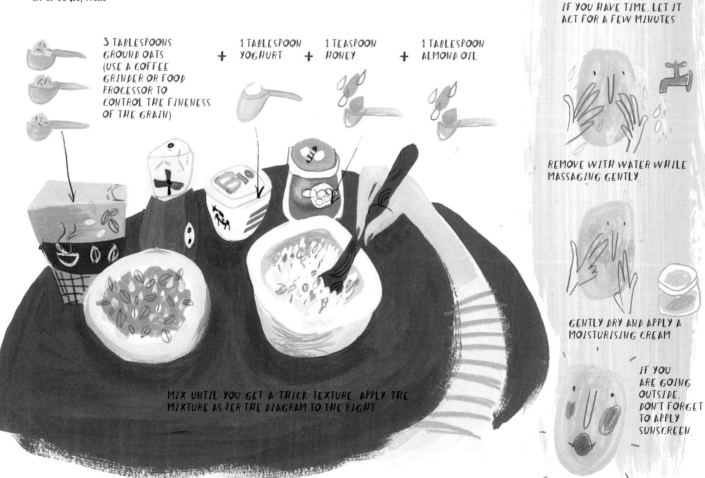

3 TABLESPOONS GROUND OATS (USE A COFFEE GRINDER OR FOOD PROCESSOR TO CONTROL THE FINENESS OF THE GRAIN)

+ 1 TABLESPOON YOGHURT

+ 1 TEASPOON HONEY

+ 1 TABLESPOON ALMOND OIL

MIX UNTIL YOU GET A THICK TEXTURE. APPLY THE MIXTURE AS PER THE DIAGRAM TO THE RIGHT

APPLY THE MIXTURE TO A SLIGHTLY DAMP FACE, AVOIDING THE EYE CONTOUR

IF YOU HAVE TIME, LET IT ACT FOR A FEW MINUTES

REMOVE WITH WATER WHILE MASSAGING GENTLY.

GENTLY DRY AND APPLY A MOISTURISING CREAM.

IF YOU ARE GOING OUTSIDE, DON'T FORGET TO APPLY SUNSCREEN.

## RICE SCRUB

Rice has many properties, but its brightening capacity stands out. You can use rice flour or grind the grains yourself in a coffee grinder. Make sure it has a smooth texture that won't harm your skin.

In a bowl, mix:

- 2 tablespoons ground rice
- 1 tablespoon coconut oil
- 1 teaspoon honey

If you want to add brightening effects, you can add a splash (just a splash!) of lemon juice, milk or yoghurt.

Mix the ingredients until you get a thick paste, as in the previous recipes. Remember not to press against the skin and moisturise thoroughly afterwards.

## COCONUT AND ALMOND SCRUB

This gentle scrub is full of nutrients and will leave you with smooth and radiant skin!

For this recipe you need unroasted sweet almonds that are as fresh as possible. Grind them to the optimum consistency, which is just before the almond meal turns into flour.

In a bowl, mix:

- 2 tablespoons ground almonds
- 2 tablespoons shredded coconut
- 1 tablespoon coconut or almond oil
- 2 tablespoons milk. For a vegan option, opt for rose water, non-dairy milk, or a chamomile infusion

## REFRESHING CUCUMBER AND ALOE SCRUB

This refreshing scrub is wonderful for the summer months or to prepare the skin before sun exposure. The soothing properties of aloe and the toning properties of cucumber will leave your skin clean and fresh.

In a bowl, mix:

- ⅓ large cucumber, chopped, but not too finely
- 1 tablespoon white sugar
- 2 tablespoons aloe vera
- 1 tablespoon yoghurt, optional

You can adapt this recipe for the whole body, adding the whole cucumber, sea salt and a drop of mint essential oil to increase the cooling sensation.

## LAVENDER AND WHITE CLAY EXFOLIATING POWDER

This wonderful facial peel will leave you with clean and renewed skin, thanks to the calming effects of lavender and the cleansing and detoxifying agents found in white clay. This preparation will keep for months in a ventilated place. In a bowl, mix:

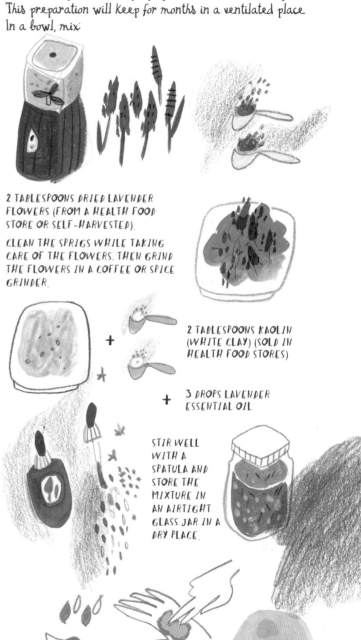

2 TABLESPOONS DRIED LAVENDER FLOWERS (FROM A HEALTH FOOD STORE OR SELF-HARVESTED).

CLEAN THE SPRIGS WHILE TAKING CARE OF THE FLOWERS, THEN GRIND THE FLOWERS IN A COFFEE OR SPICE GRINDER.

2 TABLESPOONS KAOLIN (WHITE CLAY) (SOLD IN HEALTH FOOD STORES)

3 DROPS LAVENDER ESSENTIAL OIL

STIR WELL WITH A SPATULA AND STORE THE MIXTURE IN AN AIRTIGHT GLASS JAR IN A DRY PLACE.

TO APPLY, PUT A SMALL AMOUNT IN THE PALM OF YOUR HAND AND ADD WATER OR A HYDROSOL (LAVENDER, ROSE OR WITCH-HAZEL). MIX IT WITH YOUR FINGERS UNTIL IT FORMS A PASTE, THEN APPLY AS IN THE OTHER RECIPES.

# BODY SCRUBS

## CITRUS SCRUB

The relaxing scent of citrus is invigorating and revitalising. With this sugar-based scrub, your skin will be resplendent.

You will need:

- 1 small cup brown sugar
- 4 tablespoons coconut oil
- 2 tablespoons almond oil
- 6 drops of tangerine essential oil
- zest of 1 lemon and 1 orange
- marigold flowers to decorate

Combine the oils. If the coconut oil is solid, heat it in a water bath until it melts. Add the essential oil and the citrus zests and mix thoroughly until you have a smooth paste. Stir in the marigold flowers. Store it in a glass jar in a corner of the bathroom. Apply carefully, using circular motions, avoiding delicate areas and concentrating on rough areas.

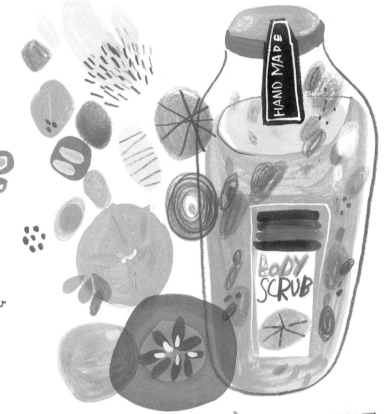

## HERB AND OLIVE OIL BODY SCRUB

The wonderful smell of this energising and refreshing scrub will transport you to a Mediterranean forest.

You will need:

- lavender flowers
- sage and thyme leaves
- 3 tablespoons olive oil
- 3 tablespoons almond oil
- 8 drops lavender essential oil
- 3 drops rosemary essential oil
- 1 small cup sea salt

Use a coffee grinder to grind the lavender flowers, thyme leaves and sage leaves. Pick over the sprigs first to remove the woody stems. Fresh lavender or rosemary flowers you have gathered would also be perfect here.

Mix the oils, then add the essential oils, salt and your ground herbs. Use the scrub and enjoy its scent!

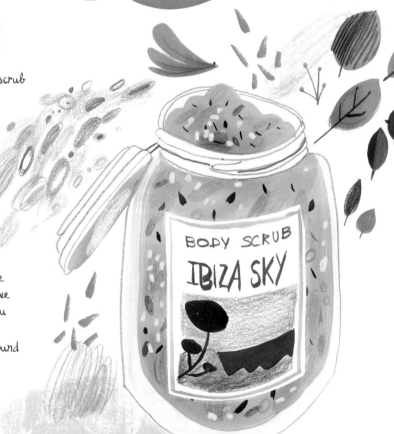

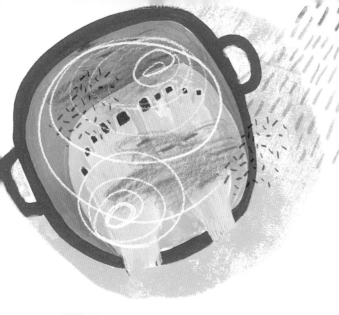

## SEA SAND FOOT SCRUB

Beach vacation? Good memories of days by the sea can come in the form of a treatment like this. Sand has an exfoliating quality that will remove dead skin and leave your feet relaxed and soft.

You will need:

- 5 tablespoons fine beach sand
- 1 tablespoon Epsom salts (or substitute sea salt)
- 1 tablespoon coconut oil
- 4 drops essential oil (tea tree, lemon or lavender)

Combine all the ingredients and gently massage the mixture onto your feet, especially the soles and heels. Let your feet rest in water for a while to benefit from the relaxing effects of the Epsom salts.

## LIP EXFOLIATOR

The soft skin of the lips deserves a gentle exfoliator. Once a month will suffice.

You will need:

- 1 tablespoon honey
- 1 tablespoon brown sugar
- ½ tablespoon almond or olive oil

Combine all the ingredients and apply to your lips with your finger, gently massaging it in. Rinse with lukewarm water and apply a moisturising balm. You can add crushed berries or a strawberry for flavour.

## COFFEE AND CINNAMON ANTI-CELLULITE EXFOLIANT

Caffeine and cinnamon have draining effects, which facilitate the elimination of toxins. In addition to exfoliating, this recipe stimulates the circulation where cellulite has accumulated. Do not apply it to sensitive skin areas.

You will need:

- 50 g ground coffee (you can recycle your used coffee grounds)
- 50 g brown sugar
- 15 g ground cinnamon
- 20 g coconut oil
- 8 drops cypress essential oil (optional)
- 8 drops ginger essential oil (optional)

Combine all the ingredients and apply the mixture to wet skin, concentrating on the hips and legs, where you have cellulite. Always massage in a circular motion from the the bottom upwards, towards the heart.

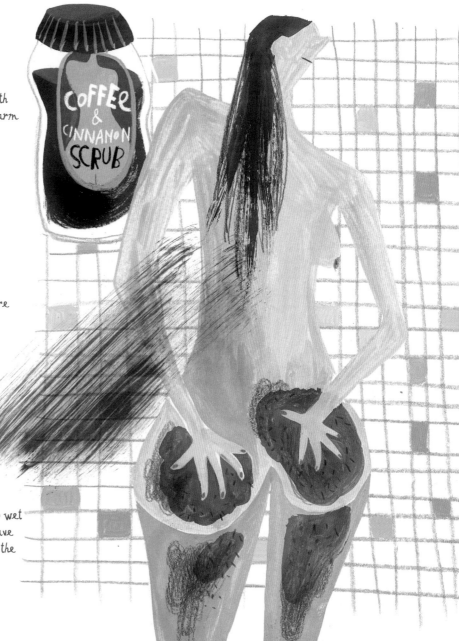

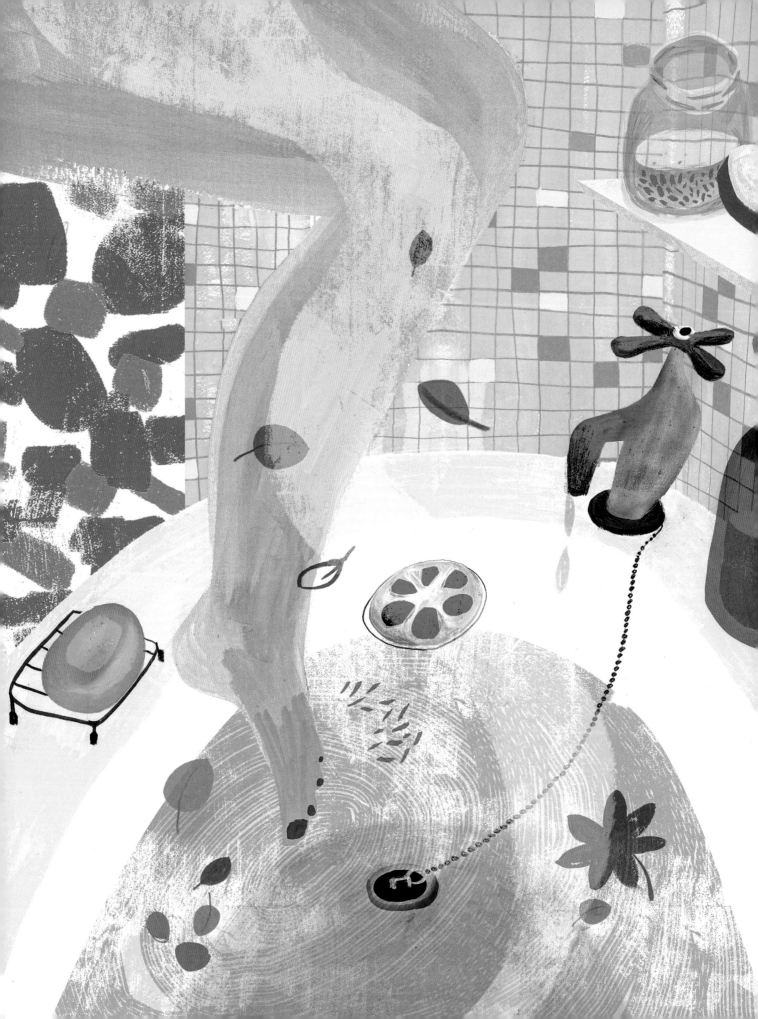

# Baths

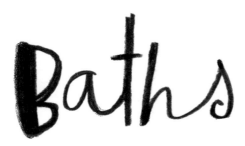

Do you feel a strong urge to disconnect and just relax? A good bath can be an excellent emergency solution for both your skin and your mind. You don't need to go to a spa to enjoy the benefits of hot water and a natural treatment, you can easily prepare it yourself with ingredients from your pantry.

Hot baths improve blood circulation, relax the muscles, clear the airways, help induce sleep, relax the mind, and cleanse and draw out impurities from the skin. A Sunday afternoon or after-work bath can be a luxurious beauty and health experience.

The ideal temperature for baths should be no higher than 37°C (99°F) and immersion should not exceed 15 or 20 minutes. During that time, you can take the opportunity to apply a facial or hair mask while you relax with your favourite playlist, meditate or share the bathroom with your partner. At the end, you can finish with a cold shower to reactivate your circulation (remember to direct the stream of water towards your heart).

Infusions and foods such as honey, milk and oatmeal will add beneficial properties to the bath water and give your skin a wonderful dose of nutrition and hydration. But the star ingredient for a relaxing bath is sea salt.

There are many different types of salt. Himalayan rose is known for its multiple therapeutic properties. Epsom salt (magnesium sulphate) comes from underground deposits, and due to its magnesium content, offers innumerable properties for the skin and the body (it exfoliates, relaxes tight muscles and detoxifies …).

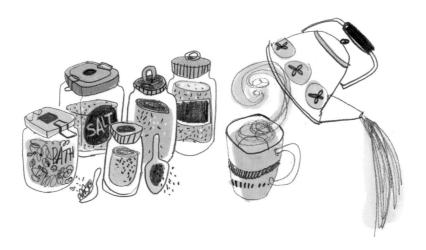

# BODY BATHS

## CLEOPATRA-STYLE NOURISHING BATH

The recipe for this wonderfully exfoliating and moisturising bath substitutes cow's milk and yoghurt for Cleopatra's donkey milk. Honey provides large amounts of minerals and nutrients, as do kaolin (white clay) and essential oils. The idea is that this soak serves as a mask and a bath at the same time. You can also apply it to the face.

In a bowl, mix:

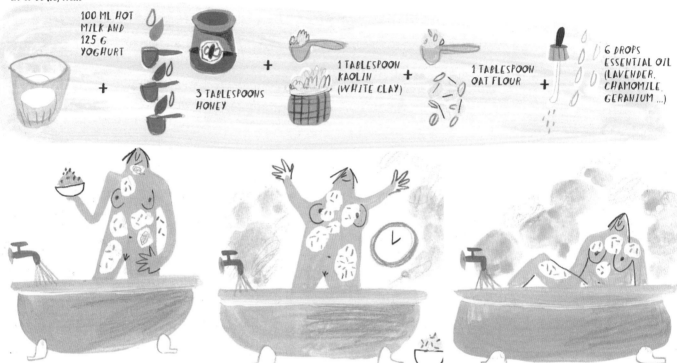

100 ML HOT MILK AND 125 G YOGHURT

+ 3 TABLESPOONS HONEY

+ 1 TABLESPOON KAOLIN (WHITE CLAY)

+ 1 TABLESPOON OAT FLOUR

+ 6 DROPS ESSENTIAL OIL (LAVENDER, CHAMOMILE, GERANIUM ...)

Stand in the bathtub, then apply the mixture all over your body and face. Let it act for a few minutes before slowly entering the water. Let 15 minutes pass then rinse all over with warm water. Dry the skin gently.

## BATH FOR SENSITIVE SKIN

This bath is for people with inflamed or sensitive skin, as well as children. It will make things much easier if you put the ingredients into a recyclable muslin bag so you can easily remove the mixture from the water when you are done. Oats are the essential ingredient - they are fantastic for irritations and dermatitis.

In a bowl, mix:

- 4 tablespoons colloidal oatmeal
- 2 tablespoons dried chamomile flowers
- 3 drops chamomile essential oil, dissolved in 1 tablespoon almond oil (optional)

Combine the ingredients and put the mixture in a bag that can be tied to the tap. Allow the hot water to run through the bag as the bath fills up, then get in and enjoy a 15-minute bath.

You can complement it with almond oil to hydrate dry areas.

## RELAXING FLORAL BATH

You can prepare this mixture in a decorative jar and store it in a dry place in the bathroom, to have it on hand at any time. It is also ideal to give as a gift! It is a fantastic recipe to help you relax after a stressful day and to ensure a good night's sleep.

In a bowl, mix (amount for 1 bath):

- 1 tablespoon Himalayan pink salt
- 2 tablespoons organic sea salt
- 1 tablespoon Epsom salts
- 1 tablespoon baking soda
- 2 tablespoons dried flowers (lavender, chamomile and marigold)
- 6 drops lavender essential oil
- 2 tablespoons powdered milk (optional)

## SEA BATH

With all the nostalgia of past vacations, this bath will transport you back to days full of sun and sea. It's perfect during hot months, as long as the water temperature is not too high.

- 2 tablespoons baking soda
- 4 tablespoons coarse sea salt
- 2 tablespoons Epsom salts
- 2 tablespoons coconut oil
- 5 tablespoons chopped seaweed (nori, chlorella, spirulina powder - whatever you have at home)

## PURIFYING BATH

This bath has purifying effects thanks to the apple cider vinegar.

- 2 tablespoons Epsom salts
- 2 tablespoons baking soda
- 5 tablespoons organic apple cider vinegar
- 1 tablespoon grated ginger
- 1 lemon, sliced, to decorate
- 5 drops lemon essential oil (but only if you are not going in the sun after bathing)

## APHRODISIAC CHOCOLATE BATH (SPECIAL COUPLES)

To the properties of chocolate for the skin, add the sensuality of cinnamon and ginger and the sweetness of honey. This bath, with its aphrodisiac properties, allows for a gentle body massage to be enjoyed later in the hot tub. The skin will be soft, glowing and very sweet!
In a bowl, mix:

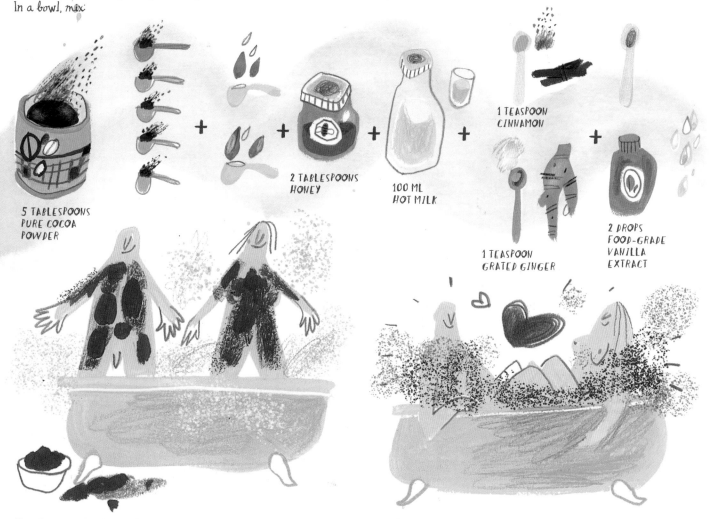

5 TABLESPOONS PURE COCOA POWDER  +  2 TABLESPOONS HONEY  +  100 ML HOT MILK  +  1 TEASPOON CINNAMON / 1 TEASPOON GRATED GINGER  +  2 DROPS FOOD-GRADE VANILLA EXTRACT

Mix the ingredients until thick, adding more milk if needed. Standing in the bathtub, rub the mixture all over your body (if you are bathing with a partner, you can apply it to each other!). Next, little by little, sink into the hot water, staying for a maximum of 15 minutes, letting the ingredients dissolve in the water.
Ideally, have some candles lit and an essential oil diffuser to fill the bathroom with the scent of cinnamon and orange.

# EFFERVESCENT BATH BOMBS

Do you have the afternoon free and feel like doing a fun craft project? Or are you looking for a gift for a friend? These effervescent bath salt bombs are good for taking care of your skin, and you'll have fun making them. In a bowl, place:

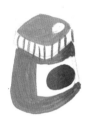 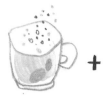 + 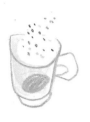 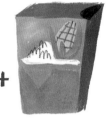 +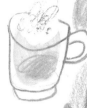

**1 SMALL CUP BAKING SODA**

**5 TABLESPOONS CITRIC ACID (CAN BE FOUND IN THE CLEANING AISLE OF SUPERMARKETS OR IN PHARMACIES)**

**5 TABLESPOONS CORNFLOUR (CORNSTARCH)**

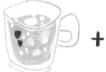 +

**5 TABLESPOONS EPSOM SALTS**

**IN A SEPARATE BOWL, MIX:**

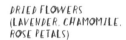

**DRIED FLOWERS (LAVENDER, CHAMOMILE, ROSE PETALS)**

COMBINE THE INGREDIENTS WELL SO THAT THEY FORM A HOMOGENEOUS MIXTURE.

**FOOD COLOURING (OPTIONAL)**

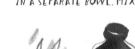 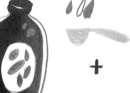 + 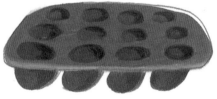 + +

**1 TABLESPOON VEGETABLE OIL**

**50 ML MINERAL WATER**

**8 DROPS ESSENTIAL OIL (YOUR CHOICE)**

ADD THE LIQUID MIXTURE TO THE SOLIDS, LITTLE BY LITTLE WHILE MIXING, TO PREVENT THE CITRIC ACID FROM REACTING.

FEEL THE DOUGH WITH YOUR HANDS. IF IT IS VERY DRY, MOISTEN IT SLIGHTLY WITH A LITTLE WATER SPRAY.

THE DOUGH SHOULD LEAVE AN INDENT WHEN PRESSED WITH YOUR FINGER, LIKE WET SAND AT THE BEACH.

POUR THE MIXTURE INTO A SILICONE MOULD (ONE FOR ICE CUBES OR CUPCAKES WILL WORK WELL). PRESS DOWN TO COMPACT THE MIXTURE.

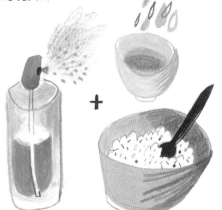 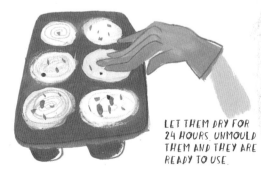 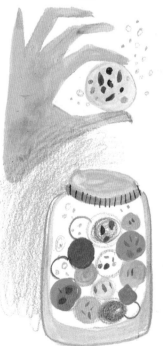

LET THEM DRY FOR 24 HOURS, UNMOULD THEM AND THEY ARE READY TO USE.

# FOOT BATHS

The feet are a forgotten part of the body and it is important to take care of them (in all seasons!). They need exfoliation and hydration and are essential to maintain our balance. Foot baths improve circulation and relieve tension and stress.

If you don't have a bathtub at home, all you need is a small basin or bucket to dip your feet in and you can achieve the same rewarding and relaxing effects as those of a full-body bath.

## FOR TIRED FEET

This is great after a tiring day. You need two basins to facilitate the temperature contrast that will help reduce the inflammation of tired feet and improve circulation.

- 1 basin of cold water
- 1 basin of hot water
- handful of chamomile and marigold flowers (or 5 drops chamomile and lavender essential oil.)
- handful of Epsom salts (or sea salt)

First, add the flowers to the basin of hot water, then put your feet in for 5 minutes. After that, put them in the basin of cold water for a few minutes (the shower jet would also work). Next, place your feet back in the basin of hot water and add the salts. Leave them there for 15 minutes. Dry well and moisturise.

## FOR BAD FOOT ODOURS

Footwear and sweaty secretions favour bacteria, which cause bad odours, and the humidity of swimming pools and gyms allows the proliferation of fungi. For both cases, this disinfectant and pH-regulating bath can be a fantastic solution.

In a bowl, mix:

- 1 small cup apple cider vinegar
- 2 tablespoons bicarb soda
- 3 drops tea tree essential oil
- 6 drops lavender essential oil

Add all the ingredients to hot water and submerge your feet for 20 minutes. Dry well and moisturise.

# SHOWER DISCS

Don't have a bathtub and want to enjoy the scents of essential oils in your daily shower instead? You can make baking soda-based discs that will release the smells of essential oils under water, and help keep your shower clean. They can be stored in a sealed container for a long time. Perfect as a gift.

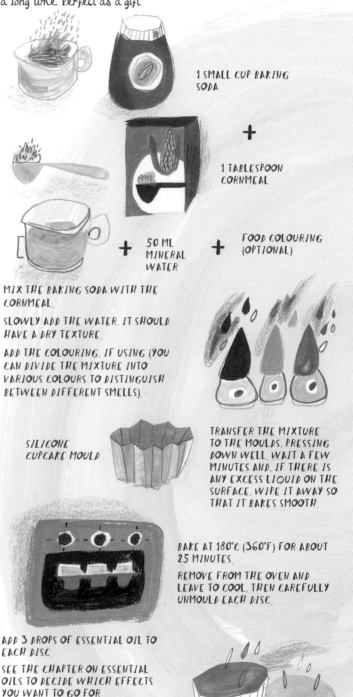

1 SMALL CUP BAKING SODA

+

1 TABLESPOON CORNMEAL

+ 50 ML MINERAL WATER

+ FOOD COLOURING (OPTIONAL)

MIX THE BAKING SODA WITH THE CORNMEAL.

SLOWLY ADD THE WATER. IT SHOULD HAVE A DRY TEXTURE.

ADD THE COLOURING, IF USING (YOU CAN DIVIDE THE MIXTURE INTO VARIOUS COLOURS TO DISTINGUISH BETWEEN DIFFERENT SMELLS).

SILICONE CUPCAKE MOULD

TRANSFER THE MIXTURE TO THE MOULDS, PRESSING DOWN WELL. WAIT A FEW MINUTES AND, IF THERE IS ANY EXCESS LIQUID ON THE SURFACE, WIPE IT AWAY SO THAT IT BAKES SMOOTH.

BAKE AT 180°C (360°F) FOR ABOUT 25 MINUTES.

REMOVE FROM THE OVEN AND LEAVE TO COOL, THEN CAREFULLY UNMOULD EACH DISC.

ADD 3 DROPS OF ESSENTIAL OIL TO EACH DISC.

SEE THE CHAPTER ON ESSENTIAL OILS TO DECIDE WHICH EFFECTS YOU WANT TO GO FOR.

WHEN YOU SHOWER, PUT A DISC ON THE FLOOR, LET THE HOT WATER PERMEATE IT AND ENJOY THE SMELL OF THE ESSENTIAL OILS.

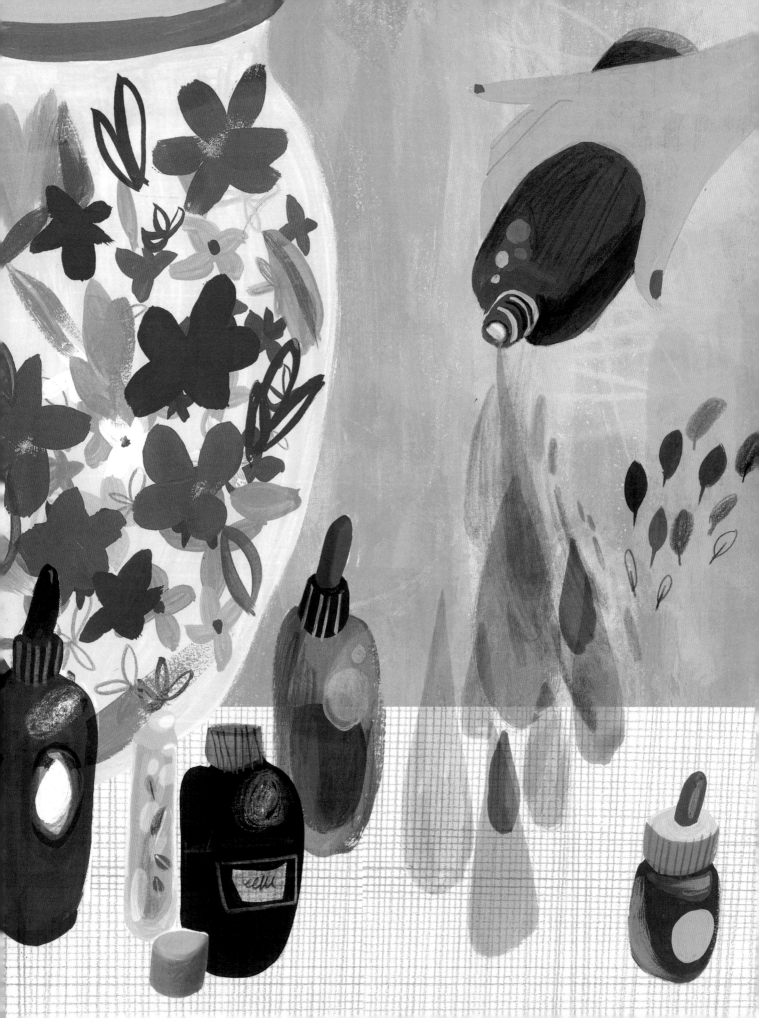

# oils and serums

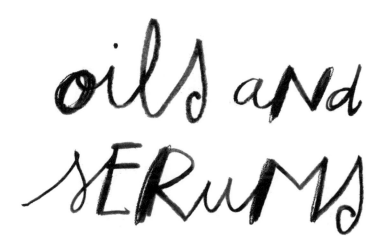

Vegetable oils are powerful cosmetics by themselves – you don't need to add anything else to take care of your skin. The goal is to find the oil that best suits your skin and, above all, to ensure that it is of the highest quality.

The alliance between essential oils and vegetable oils offers many possibilities, since it allows us to personalise our skin care based on the characteristics of our skin and our preferred scents.

If you're used to conventional creams, you might be a little scared to apply an oil, perhaps thinking that it will leave your skin too oily. On the contrary – the oil will be absorbed by your skin, nourishing it deeply. Some oils, such as jojoba, even have the ability to balance excess fat.

Oil can draw dirt from the skin without clogging the pores, so it is also ideal for removing make-up and cleansing the skin before bed. However, you should still be aware of the comedogenic level (that is, the likelihood that a substance will clog pores) of the oils you use if you are prone to acne. The lowest are argan, shea butter, castor oil, jojoba, apricot kernel, grape seed and rosehip. Among the highest are wheatgerm oil and coconut oil.

One of the strengths of skincare products made from vegetable oils is that we can enrich their properties by adding essential oils (don't confuse them!) or infusing them with plants to create serums and massage oils. We can also use them as base ingredients to make balms, creams and soaps.

Although they have a fairly long shelf life, it is important to use them as soon as possible, keep them in cool places during the summer months and protect them from light. It is also important to store them in opaque glass containers. It is helpful to add vitamin E (which is also beneficial for your skin) to prevent oxidation and prolong their shelf life. You can find vitamin E in drops or capsules, as it is also used as a food supplement.

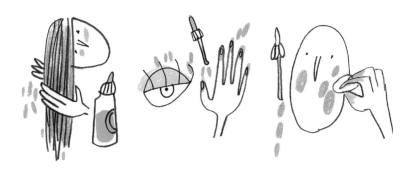

# FACIAL CLEANSING WITH VEGETABLE OILS

The oil cleansing method works very well for all skin types. A mixture of well-selected oils is ideal for cleansing, removing make-up and regulating oil in the skin. Vegetable oils help dissolve and remove toxins and impurities embedded in the pores. Castor oil is often used as a base due to its antibacterial properties, but any oil will work if you choose one that's right for your skin type. I recommend that you try the method described below for a couple of weeks.

It is important to use clean, recyclable pads or towels for each application, as this will help keep the oil pure and clean.

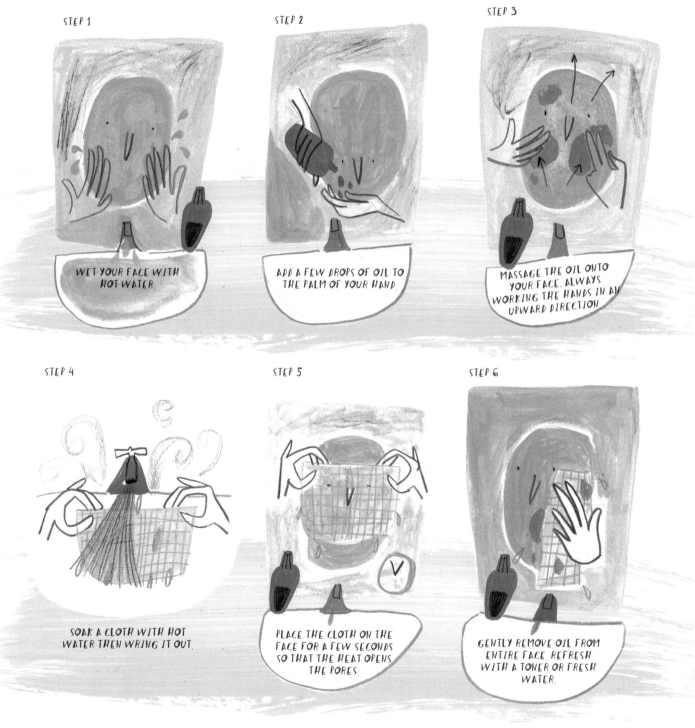

STEP 1
WET YOUR FACE WITH HOT WATER.

STEP 2
ADD A FEW DROPS OF OIL TO THE PALM OF YOUR HAND.

STEP 3
MASSAGE THE OIL ONTO YOUR FACE. ALWAYS WORKING THE HANDS IN AN UPWARD DIRECTION.

STEP 4
SOAK A CLOTH WITH HOT WATER THEN WRING IT OUT.

STEP 5
PLACE THE CLOTH ON THE FACE FOR A FEW SECONDS SO THAT THE HEAT OPENS THE PORES.

STEP 6
GENTLY REMOVE OIL FROM ENTIRE FACE. REFRESH WITH A TONER OR FRESH WATER.

# VEGETABLE OIL AND ESSENTIAL OIL ACCORDING TO YOUR SKIN TYPE

Use the table below as a guide for combining your vegetable and essential oils. You should not add essential oils to cleaning treatments, as they can irritate the eyes. Use these instructions for combinations to make serums, creams or elixirs. The dilution of essential oil in carrier oil must be between 1% and 2.5% of the total preparation.

You must use essential oils with caution, a few drops is enough to benefit from their properties. Remember that citrus fruits (bergamot, lemon, tangerine etc..) are photosensitive and can react with sunlight.

| SKIN TYPE | NORMAL | DRY | OILY | MIXED | SENSITIVE | MATURE | ACNEIC |
|---|---|---|---|---|---|---|---|
| VEGETABLE OIL | jojoba, olive, grape seed, almond, argan, coconut, castor, hazelnut | almond, avocado, rosehip, wheatgerm, argan, coconut, apricot kernel, jojoba, olive, grape seed | jojoba, sesame, castor, grape seed, hazelnut | jojoba, grape seed, hazelnut, olive, argan, sesame | almond, argan, hazelnut, rosehip, evening primrose, olive, sesame | rosehip, almond, avocado, coconut, argan, olive, wheatgerm, hazelnut | jojoba, evening primrose, sesame, grape seed, castor |
| ESSENTIAL OIL | lavender, chamomile, rosewood, geranium, neroli, ylang ylang, damask rose | chamomile, incense, rosewood, jasmine, geranium, neroli, ylang ylang, damask rose | bergamot, cedar, cypress, lemon, frankincense, sage, thyme, rock rose | lavender, bergamot, patchouli, cedar, geranium | chamomile, lavender, jasmine, neroli | frankincense, lavender, ylang ylang, neroli, rosewood, sandalwood, damask rose, sage | tea tree, lavender, thyme, geranium |

## CLEANSING WITH CASTOR OIL

Castor oil is the ideal base for the oil cleansing method thanks to its antibacterial and anti-inflammatory properties. To lighten its thick consistency, mix it with other oils that work well for your skin type. The approximate ratios are:

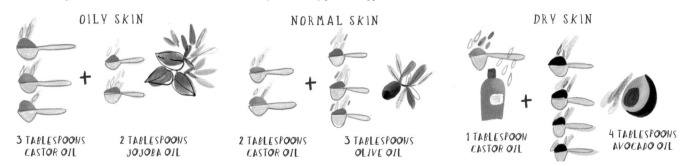

**OILY SKIN**
3 TABLESPOONS CASTOR OIL + 2 TABLESPOONS JOJOBA OIL

**NORMAL SKIN**
2 TABLESPOONS CASTOR OIL + 3 TABLESPOONS OLIVE OIL

**DRY SKIN**
1 TABLESPOON CASTOR OIL + 4 TABLESPOONS AVOCADO OIL

Store the mixture in an opaque glass bottle, and add a few drops of vitamin E to prevent it going rancid.
Apply it using the oil cleansing method shown opposite.

# FACIAL OILS

Facial oils work perfectly as treatment serums. The benefits of vegetable oil are mixed with those of essential oils. Take care not to fill storage jars to the top - it's important to leave a little space to stir the mixture. Ideally, use it before going to bed and massage into the face well, which will help tone facial muscles and facilitate absorption.

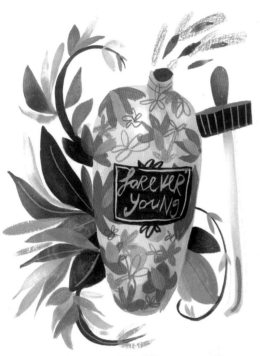

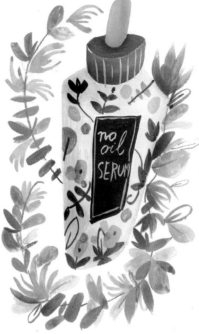

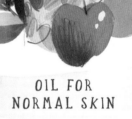

### OIL FOR MATURE SKIN

This blend of oils is a powerful antioxidant and anti-wrinkle cream.

- 1 tablespoon evening primrose oil
- 1 tablespoon argan oil
- 2 tablespoons jojoba oil
- 1 teaspoon rosehip oil
- 3 drops vitamin E
- 2 drops palmarosa essential oil
- 2 drops frankincense essential oil
- 2 drops neroli essential oil

### OIL FOR OILY SKIN

Jojoba oil is the most suitable for oily skin, as it is balancing and quickly absorbed.

- 2 tablespoons jojoba oil
- 1 tablespoon apricot oil
- 3 drops vitamin E
- 3 drops tea tree essential oil
- 3 drops ylang ylang essential oil

### OIL FOR NORMAL SKIN

This oil is great to take with you when you travel, as it can be used for hair, hands, nails, face and feet. It's a perfect mix for normal or combination skin.

- 2 tablespoons jojoba oil
- 2 tablespoons almond oil
- 2 tablespoons apricot oil
- 6 drops vitamin E
- 3 drops geranium essential oil
- 3 drops lavender essential oil

### EYE CONTOUR OIL

The mixture of these oils hydrates, protects and nourishes the skin area around the eyes.
Do not add essential oils.
In a 15 ml roll-on or dropper bottle, mix:

1 TEASPOON ARGAN OIL

+

1 TEASPOON WHEATGERM OIL

+

1 TEASPOON AVOCADO OIL

+

1 DROP VITAMIN E

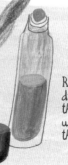

Roll on or apply small drops around the eye, then gently massage using small touches with the tips of your fingers.

# MACERATED OILS

## MULTIPURPOSE MACERATED OIL

You can use this oil as a cleanser, facial and body moisturiser, for children, after sun exposure (mixed with aloe), for irritations, flaking, itches, for making balms, creams, soaps ... It's worth finding a good quality oil and making a mash like this!

The chapter on preparations with plants (page 26) explains how to prepare an oil macerate. For this recipe, you will need:

- lavender flowers
- marigold flowers
- chamomile flowers
- olive oil or sweet almond oil

Take a jar that has been sterilised and disinfected with alcohol, and fill it with a mix of flowers. Add oil until it covers the flowers completely, not leaving much room at the top. Cover the opening with plastic wrap or parchment paper, so that any potential rust from the lid never gets into the oil. Close it tightly and place it in an outdoor place, where it gets some sun during the day and is exposed to the changes in temperature (for example, a balcony). Stir it periodically, then after 40 days strain it well. It's then ready to use.

Store it in a dry, dark place and label it with the date and ingredients.

If you are short on time, you can put the jar in a water bath for 2 hours over very low heat (hot maceration), or place it in the dishwasher on a long cycle set to about 40°C (104°F). It's not the same, but it works.

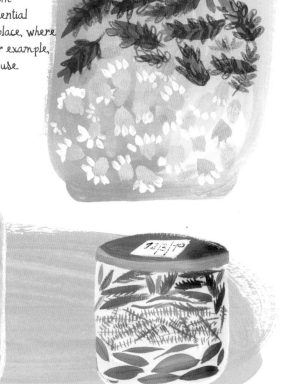

## MACERATION FOR BUMPS AND TIGHT MUSCLES

Arnica and hypericum are plants recommended for blows, bruises or tight muscles. Use this ancient and classic combination as an oil, or to make ointments or balms. Remember that St John's Wort is photosensitising - do not use it when the skin will be exposed to the sun.

- arnica flowers
- St John's wort flowers

## BETA-CAROTENE MACERATION

Fantastic for skin and hair. The beta-carotene content makes it an ideal oil to prepare the skin for summer, preserve a tan and prevent aging. Add it to your creams, ointments and soaps. To make it, place some washed and well-dried carrots into a glass jar, and continue as above.

## HAIR MACERATION

For an oil full of hair strengthening properties and to prevent hair loss, use the following plants:

- nettle leaves
- rosemary
- bay leaves

Use for hair massages, mix it in lotions or add it to your usual shampoo.

# BODY OILS

## AROMATHERAPY MASSAGE OIL

A relaxing massage is always a great beauty treatment, and by combining its effects with the hydration of vegetable oil and aromatherapy, we get all possible benefits. See the box on page 52 about the positive effects essential oils can have on your emotions. Here are some ideas:

### FOR LOVERS
6 TABLESPOONS VEGETABLE OIL
15 DROPS TANGERINE ESSENTIAL OIL
5 DROPS YLANG YLANG ESSENTIAL OIL
5 DROPS FRANKINCENSE ESSENTIAL OIL

### MUSCLE RELAXANT
3 TABLESPOONS ARNICA OIL
3 TABLESPOONS VEGETABLE OIL
8 DROPS ROSEMARY ESSENTIAL OIL
15 DROPS LAVENDER ESSENTIAL OIL

### CONCENTRATION
6 TABLESPOONS VEGETABLE OIL
8 DROPS ROSEMARY ESSENTIAL OIL
8 DROPS LEMON ESSENTIAL OIL
6 DROPS CEDAR ESSENTIAL OIL
3 DROPS MINT ESSENTIAL OIL

### FOR SLEEP
6 TABLESPOONS VEGETABLE OIL
10 DROPS LAVENDER ESSENTIAL OIL
8 DROPS CHAMOMILE ESSENTIAL OIL
6 DROPS PETITGRAIN OR MANDARIN ESSENTIAL OIL

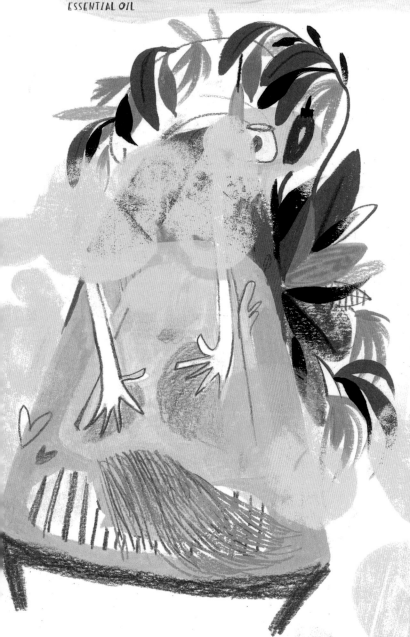

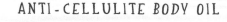

## ANTI-CELLULITE BODY OIL

Ingredients to make a draining anti-cellulite oil and for tired legs:

- 2 tablespoons calophylle vegetable oil
- 1 tablespoon almond oil
- 10 drops vitamin E
- 6 drops cypress essential oil
- 4 drops rosemary essential oil
- 2 drops peppermint essential oil

## MOISTURISING BODY OIL

This oil is perfect for after showering, waxing, etc.

- 2 tablespoons apricot oil
- 2 tablespoons jojoba oil
- 2 tablespoons almond oil (or use the macerated flower oil from page 87)
- 10 drops vitamin E
- 8 drops lavender essential oil
- 4 drops chamomile essential oil

## AFTER SUN BODY OIL

This oil is repairing and calming.

- 2 tablespoons coconut oil
- 2 tablespoons sesame oil
- 2 tablespoons apricot kernel oil (or use the macerated beta-carotene oil from page 87)
- 10 drops vitamin E
- 8 drops carrot essential oil
- 4 drops chamomile essential oil

## EXPRESS OIL FOR HANDS

In the kitchen, after peeling potatoes or artichokes or washing the dishes, if you don't have cream at hand, this solution is quick and super-effective.

- olive oil
- ½ lemon

Grease your hands with olive oil and rub the lemon all over them, pushing your fingers into the pulp. The lemon disinfects, brightens and softens the cuticles while the olive oil protects the nails and hydrates the hands.

## NAIL AND CUTICLE OIL

This mixture will care for and protect your hands and nails. Massage well into the cuticles so that the oil penetrates.

- 2 tablespoons olive oil
- 1 tablespoon jojoba oil
- 5 drops lemon essential oil
- 2 drops tea tree essential oil

## PIMP YOUR MASCARA

Extend the life of your mascara and get an eyelash treatment at the same time. You need:

- 1 teaspoon castor oil
- 5 drops vitamin E
- ½ teaspoon aloe vera

In a small sterilised bowl, mix the ingredients then use a dropper or pipette to add it to your tube of mascara. Use the brush to mix well.

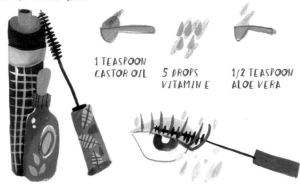

1 TEASPOON CASTOR OIL    5 DROPS VITAMIN E    1/2 TEASPOON ALOE VERA

## EYELASH AND EYEBROW OIL

Mix this treatment oil in a small bottle and apply it with a cotton pad to the eyelashes and eyelids, with the eye closed, every night before going to sleep.

- 2 tablespoons castor oil
- 2 tablespoons olive oil
- 1 tablespoon coconut oil
- a few drops vitamin E

## BEARD AND MOUSTACHE OIL

This nourishing oil will leave you with a shiny, healthy beard, and a wonderful scent. Apply it when you get out of the shower when combing your beard and moustache. You will need:

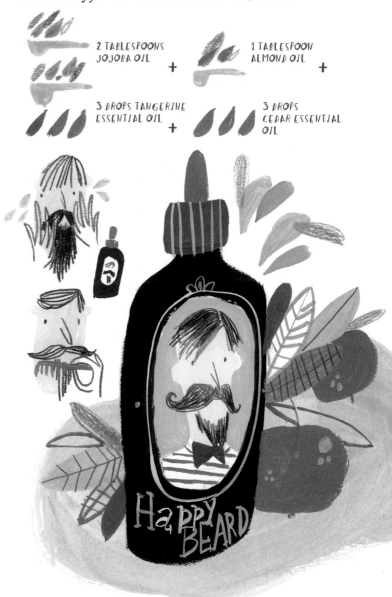

2 TABLESPOONS JOJOBA OIL + 1 TABLESPOON ALMOND OIL +

3 DROPS TANGERINE ESSENTIAL OIL + 3 DROPS CEDAR ESSENTIAL OIL

HAPPY BEARD

## HAIR OIL FOR DAMAGED ENDS

You can apply this oil as a mask before washing or as a styling serum. Apply a few drops to the palm of your hand, then distribute it from mid-lengths to ends.

- 2 tablespoons argan oil
- 2 tablespoons jojoba oil
- 2 tablespoons coconut oil
- 5 drops vitamin E
- 5 drops geranium essential oil
- 2 drops ylang ylang essential oil

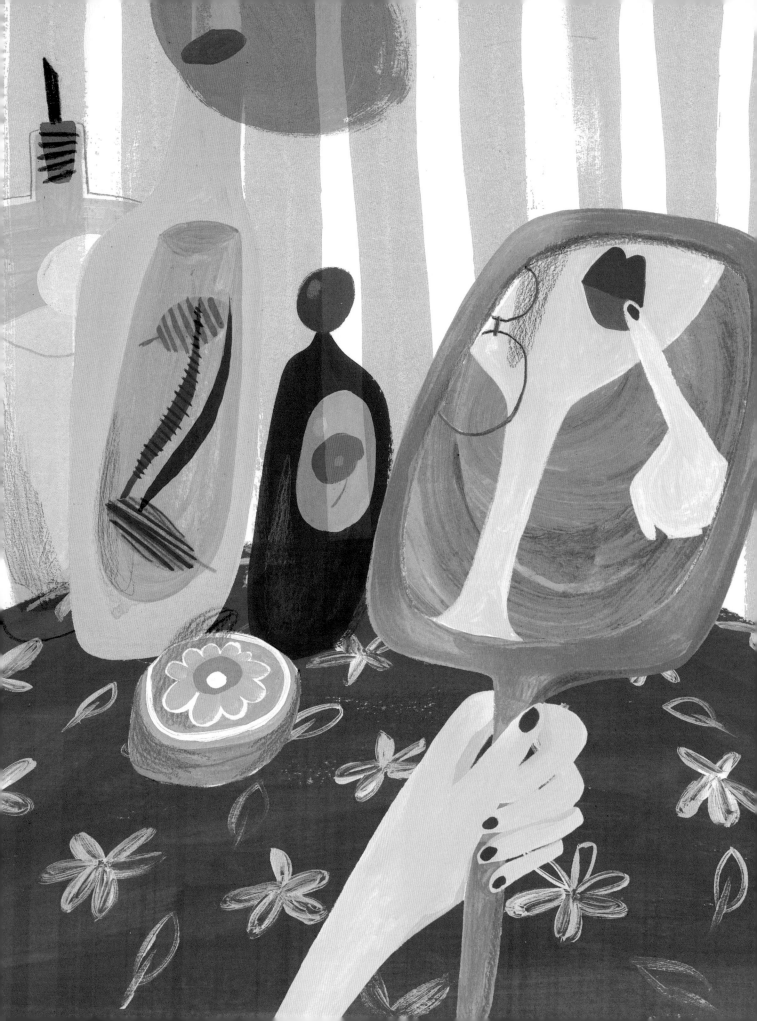

# BALMS AND BUTTERS

The word 'balm' comes from 'balsam', a tree whose aromatic resin was highly prized in Ancient Greece. Today, we associate the term with something soft that takes care of and protects us. In skin care, we use the word balm to describe mixtures with a greasy and unctuous texture whose function is to repair, protect and nourish. They are very easy to make and fantastic for the skin.

The common characteristic of these mixtures is that they are mostly composed of oils, fats and vegetable waxes. The method is very simple – it consists of melting the ingredients in a bain-marie, mixing them well and letting them cool until they solidify.

When melting, be careful not to exceed 70°C (158°F), because anything above that can destroy the beneficial properties. It is also necessary to add vitamin E (tocopherol), which, in addition to enriching the mixture due to its antioxidant properties, will help to preserve it. The vitamin E must be added at the last moment, when the fat temperatures have dropped, just before pouring the balm into a container. We do the same with essential oils, but incorporate them at the last minute due to their sensitivity to heat. The balms have a shelf life of between 6 and 12 months.

If you are used to conventional cosmetics, you will discover different textures. Vegetable fats and shortenings are absorbed more slowly and you may feel a thicker, greasy sensation. This creaminess is good for your skin: the balm will be absorbed little by little and your skin will be restored and protected.

It is also important to keep in mind that 100% natural raw materials will be affected by changes in air temperature, especially if you use coconut oil, which solidifies when cold. Keep in mind that if you live in a very cold or very hot area, you will need to slightly adjust the formulas by adding more or less liquid or solid fats.

Give yourself a hug with fats and butters – it will be wonderful!

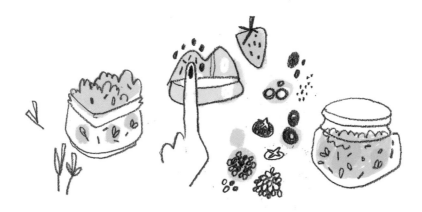

# STEP-BY-STEP: BALMS

Although preparing balms is very simple, here is a step-by-step description of the basic procedure, which you can apply to the recipes that follow. You will need a precision scale (most precision scales have the option to weigh in both imperial and metric units), a beaker or other heat-resistant container, a stirrer or spatula, a pot and bowl to make a bain-marie, a kitchen thermometer, a spoon, jars to pack the balms into and labels to record the date they are made and names.

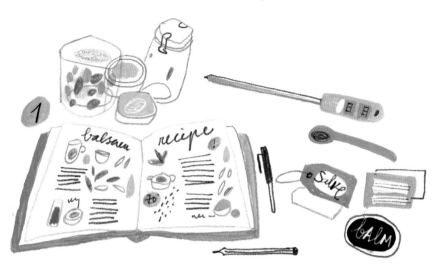

PREPARE BY ORGANISING YOUR INGREDIENTS AND WORKSPACE, WHICH MUST BE CLEAN AND DISINFECTED WITH ALCOHOL. I RECOMMEND YOU HAVE A NOTEBOOK FOR RECORDING YOUR OBSERVATIONS.

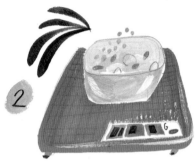

WEIGH THE INGREDIENTS. START WITH THE BEESWAX AND COCOA BUTTER. BREAK THEM INTO SMALL PIECES TO HELP THEM MELT MORE EASILY. PLACE THEM IN THE HEAT-RESISTANT CONTAINER.

ADD ALL THE OTHER INGREDIENTS (FOR EXAMPLE VITAMIN E, GLYCERINE, HONEY, ESSENTIAL OILS AND COCOA) ONCE THE FATS HAVE MELTED.

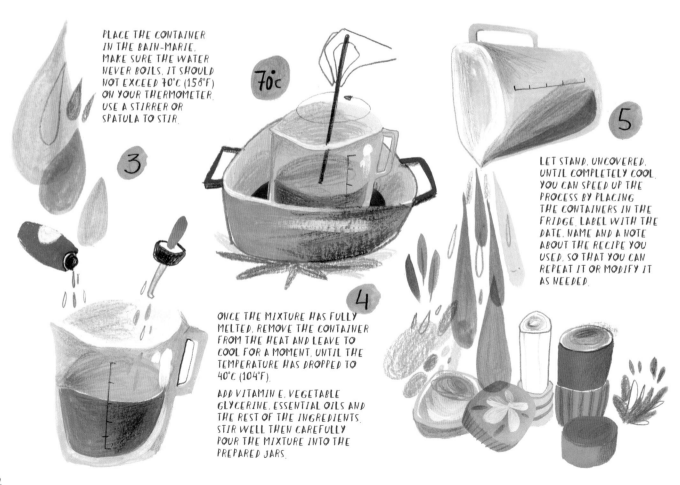

PLACE THE CONTAINER IN THE BAIN-MARIE. MAKE SURE THE WATER NEVER BOILS. IT SHOULD NOT EXCEED 70°C (158°F) ON YOUR THERMOMETER. USE A STIRRER OR SPATULA TO STIR.

70°C

ONCE THE MIXTURE HAS FULLY MELTED, REMOVE THE CONTAINER FROM THE HEAT AND LEAVE TO COOL FOR A MOMENT, UNTIL THE TEMPERATURE HAS DROPPED TO 40°C (104°F).

ADD VITAMIN E, VEGETABLE GLYCERINE, ESSENTIAL OILS AND THE REST OF THE INGREDIENTS. STIR WELL THEN CAREFULLY POUR THE MIXTURE INTO THE PREPARED JARS.

LET STAND, UNCOVERED, UNTIL COMPLETELY COOL. YOU CAN SPEED UP THE PROCESS BY PLACING THE CONTAINERS IN THE FRIDGE. LABEL WITH THE DATE, NAME AND A NOTE ABOUT THE RECIPE YOU USED, SO THAT YOU CAN REPEAT IT OR MODIFY IT AS NEEDED.

# LIP BALMS

Lip balms are the stars of homemade cosmetics. It's a good idea to start with a balm recipe, because they are easy, fun, cheap and fantastic for your wonderful lips. They also moisturise the nose and other dry areas of the body.
You can put balms in glass or plastic bottles. There are super-convenient containers for lipsticks that you can buy online, and cute little boxes made of stainless steel. If you want, add some colouring, food essence or essential oil (a couple of drops will be more than enough). As lip balms will be in contact with the mouth, we want them to be as 'edible' as possible. Before starting, remember to wash your hands well, and sterilise and disinfect utensils and containers with alcohol. You can modify the recipes according to your tastes. Play and have fun!

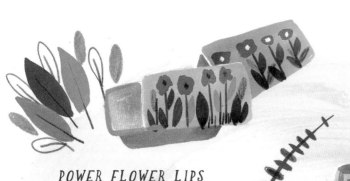

## CHOCODROPS

With a light touch of colour and the wonderful flavours of chocolate and cinnamon (makes approx. 25 g).

- 6 g coconut oil
- 5 g shea butter
- 5 g almond oil
- 5 g unrefined beeswax
- 3 g cocoa butter
- 5 drops liquid glycerine (optional)
- 2 drops vitamin E
- 1 teaspoon cocoa
- ½ teaspoon ground cinnamon

## POWER FLOWER LIPS

For dry and damaged lips. Castor oil and macerated olive oil add soothing and regenerating properties (makes approx. 25 g).

- 8 g cocoa butter
- 6 g olive oil macerated with chamomile and marigold
- 6 g castor oil
- 4 g unrefined beeswax
- 5 drops liquid glycerine (optional)
- 2 drops vitamin E
- 2 drops chamomile essential oil (optional)

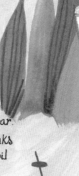

## STICK POWER

Fantastic when made as a bar. With light sun protection, thanks to shea butter and sesame oil (makes approx. 25 g).

- 10 g shea butter
- 6 g sesame oil
- 5 g cocoa butter
- 4 g unrefined beeswax
- 2 drops vitamin E
- 2 drops liquid glycerine (optional)
- 2 drops lavender essential oil (optional)

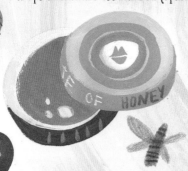

## A TASTE OF HONEY

Sweet lips and honey kisses. With almond oil to repair (makes approx. 25 g).

- 8 g cocoa butter
- 10 g almond oil
- 5 g honey
- 3 g unrefined beeswax
- 5 drops liquid glycerine (optional)
- 2 drops vitamin E

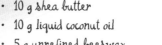

## KISS ME COCONUT!

Soft kisses and the shine of love. With shea and coconut oil (makes approx. 25 g).

- 10 g shea butter
- 10 g liquid coconut oil
- 5 g unrefined beeswax
- 2 drops vitamin E
- 2 drops orange essential oil (optional)

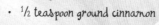

## BEAUTY OF THE NILE
### HONEY AND OLIVE CREAM

This cream is an adaptation of a traditional recipe used by the Ancient Egyptians. It is a multipurpose balm that works for everything: hands, face, stretch marks, etc. For this recipe, use a small heat-resistant glass bowl. You will also need a small hand whisk, a small silicone spatula and a sterilised 50 ml (3¼ fl oz) container.

### INGREDIENTS

- 42 g olive oil (even better is a marigold macerated oil)
- 12 g unrefined beeswax
- 8 g honey
- 10 drops liquid glycerine
- 4 drops vitamin E
- 3 drops frankincense essential oil
- 3 drops damask rose or geranium essential oil

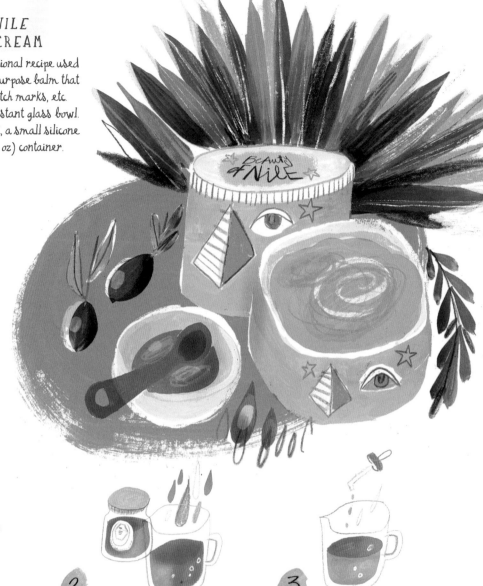

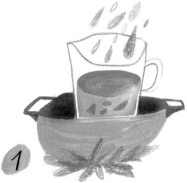

**1** WEIGH THE OLIVE OIL AND BEESWAX (REMEMBER TO CUT THE BEESWAX INTO SMALL PIECES). PUT THEM IN THE HEAT-RESISTANT BOWL THEN PUT THE BOWL IN A BAIN-MARIE.

**2** STIR WITHOUT STOPPING UNTIL THE WAX HAS MELTED INTO THE OIL. REMOVE FROM THE HEAT. WAIT FOR THE TEMPERATURE TO DROP SLIGHTLY THEN ADD THE HONEY, CONTINUING TO MIX UNTIL WELL INCORPORATED.

**3** ADD THE LIQUID GLYCERINE, THE VITAMIN E AND THE ESSENTIAL OILS. KEEP STIRRING THEN PLACE THE MIXTURE IN THE FRIDGE OR FREEZER.

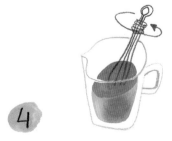

**4** AFTER A FEW MINUTES, WHEN IT STARTS TO COOL (THE EDGES SHOULD BE HARD, BUT THE MIDDLE IS STILL COMPLETELY LIQUID), REMOVE FROM THE FRIDGE AND START TO WHISK IT, SLOWLY, WITHOUT STOPPING.

YOU WILL SEE THE CREAM BEGIN TO LIGHTEN AND TAKE ON A CREAMY CONSISTENCY. ENSURE YOU STIR LITTLE BY LITTLE. IF YOU THINK IT'S NECESSARY, PUT THE CREAM BACK IN THE FRIDGE FOR A FEW MORE MINUTES UNTIL IT'S COLD.

DECANT THE CREAM INTO A CONTAINER WITH THE SILICONE SPATULA.

LABEL WITH DATE AND NAME.

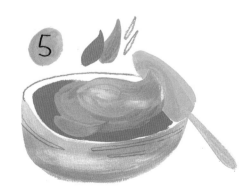

**5**

## YLANG YLANG FLOWER HAIR CREAM FOR DAMAGED ENDS

This cream is fantastic for moisturising the ends of your hair and also to set hair curls. All ingredients are protective and moisturising. Take a very small amount, rub it into your hands and apply it to the ends of your hair. You can also apply it at night before bed as a leave-in treatment. The essential oil of ylang ylang is relaxing and good for strengthening hair.

### INGREDIENTS

- 18 g shea butter
- 15 g coconut oil
- 10 g castor oil
- 6 g cocoa butter
- 5 drops liquid glycerine
- 4 drops vitamin E
- 4 drops ylang ylang essential oil

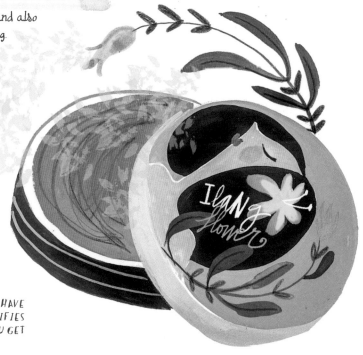

THE METHOD IS THE SAME AS IN THE PREVIOUS RECIPE. ONCE YOU HAVE THE MIXTURE READY, PUT IT IN THE FRIDGE AND, WHEN IT SOLIDIFIES AT THE EDGES, BEGIN TO BEAT UNTIL THE MIXTURE CLEARS AND YOU GET A CLEAR AND CREAMY TEXTURE.

## BALMS WITH INFUSED OILS

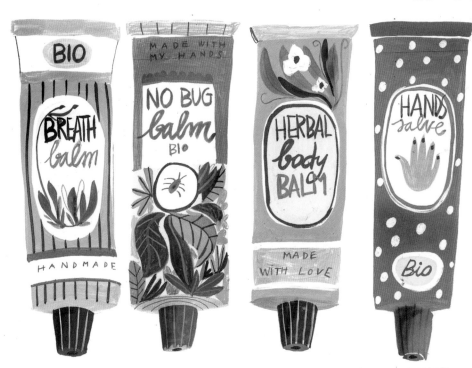

Use this recipe as a base and adapt it for different things, modifying the combinations of macerated and essential oils as desired. The method is the basic one: melt the fats and oils, then add the essential oils and vitamin E. Don't forget to write down the date and ingredients.

### FOR DRY AND DAMAGED HANDS AND SKIN

- 30 g shea butter
- 3 g beeswax
- 15 g macerated marigold and chamomile oil
- 4 drops vitamin E
- 6 drops lavender essential oil
- 6 drops chamomile essential oil

### TO BREATHE BETTER

The same proportions of lavender macerated oil mixed with pine, mint and eucalyptus essential oils.

### FOR INSECT BITES

Oil macerated with lavender, marigold and chamomile flowers combined with essential oils of tea tree, eucalyptus and lavender. It works to both drive away insects and relieve pain from their bites.

### FOR BUMPS AND TIGHT MUSCLES

The same proportions of arnica macerated oil and rosemary and eucalyptus essential oils.

# SOLID MOISTURISERS

Solid cosmetics are great for travelling and save on packaging. Use solid butters as moisturisers, for massages, as perfume or to enrich your baths … Feel how they slowly melt with the heat of your skin.

For these recipes, you need silicone moulds - the ones for ice cubes, chocolates or cupcakes work perfectly. Make sure they fit in your hand and have smooth shapes. I personally like to keep them natural, but this method allows you to play with your imagination: you can add a drop of colouring or flavouring (vanilla essence, cinnamon, orange, cocoa, dried flowers) or some type of dry seed (that have soft shapes) such as adzukis or poppy seeds.

## MOISTURISING

(Remember that you can adapt the formula based on your tastes or time of year)

- 4 g beeswax
- 42 g cocoa butter
- 12 g almond oil
- 12 g shea butter
- 15 drops vitamin E
- 20 drops essential oil of your choosing

## PERFUMES/ESSENCES

This recipe is for a harder end product, which is ideal for solid perfumes. You can fill an old lipstick container for easy storage (but don't use these on your lips). Consult the essential oils chapter to help you decide which essential oils to use.

- 30 g beeswax
- 30 g cocoa butter
- 30 g coconut oil
- 6 drops vitamin E
- 30 drops essential oil of your choosing

## FOR THE BATH

This one is made with a base of cocoa butter since it melts between 35 and 38°C (95 and 100°F). Add to bath water for fragrant hydration.

- 130 g cocoa butter
- 2 g almond oil
- flower petals
- 20 drops essential oil of your choosing

WASH THEN DISINFECT THE UTENSILS AND MOULDS YOU WILL BE USING WITH ALCOHOL, THEN WEIGH THE INGREDIENTS.

CUT THE BEESWAX INTO SMALL PIECES THEN MELT IN A HEAT-RESISTANT BOWL OVER A BAIN-MARIE. LITTLE BY LITTLE, ADD THE BUTTERS. STIR WITH A SPATULA UNTIL EVERYTHING HAS COMPLETELY MELTED.

REMOVE THE BOWL FROM THE HEAT WITHOUT STIRRING. ADD THE REST OF THE INGREDIENTS (VITAMIN E, ESSENTIAL OILS, DRIED FLOWERS, ETC.). FILL THE MOULD WITH THE MIXTURE, THEN TRANSFER TO THE FRIDGE TO COOL. IT WILL LOOK SMOOTH AND BRIGHT.

WHEN IT HAS COMPLETELY COOLED, YOUR BARS ARE READY TO USE.

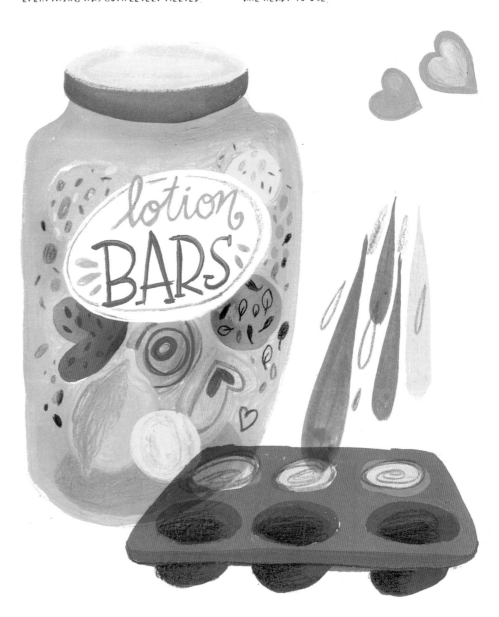

# BODY BUTTERS

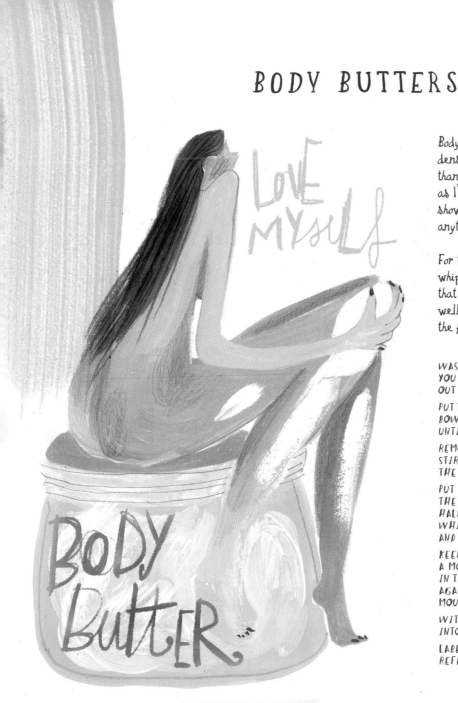

Body butters are body moisturisers that are dense and greasy, and have a thicker texture than a cream or lotion. I can't do without them, as I've gotten used to massaging my body after showering, and I wouldn't change that feeling for anything. Try it, hug yourself and you will see!

For this recipe, you need a mixer with a whipping attachment and a circular bowl that allows you to beat the mixture really well. It's about introducing air while mixing the fats to achieve a mousse-like texture.

WASH THEN DISINFECT THE UTENSILS AND MOULDS YOU WILL BE USING WITH ALCOHOL, THEN WEIGH OUT THE INGREDIENTS.

PUT THE BUTTERS IN A HEAT-RESISTANT BOWL, SET THE BOWL OVER A BAIN-MARIE AND STIR THE CONTENTS UNTIL THEY HAVE COMPLETELY MELTED.

REMOVE THE BOWL FROM THE HEAT, CONTINUE TO STIR UNTIL THE TEMPERATURE DROPS, THEN ADD THE THE ESSENTIAL OILS AND VITAMIN E.

PUT THE BOWL IN THE FRIDGE. WHEN YOU SEE THAT THE MIXTURE HAS BEGUN TO SOLIDIFY (IT CAN TAKE HALF AN HOUR OR MORE), TAKE IT OUT AND START WHIPPING IN THE MIXER. IT WILL BEGIN TO WHITEN AND TAKE ON A CREAMY APPEARANCE.

KEEP BEATING UNTIL YOU SEE THAT IT THICKENS LIKE A MOUSSE. IF NEEDED, YOU CAN PUT THE BOWL BACK IN THE FRIDGE, WAIT ABOUT 10 MINUTES, THEN WHIP AGAIN, SO THAT IT SOLIDIFIES WELL AND HOLDS THE MOUSSE-LIKE TEXTURE.

WITH A SILICONE SPATULA, TRANSFER THE MIXTURE INTO A BEAUTIFUL GLASS JAR.

LABEL THE JAR WITH THE NAME, DATE AND A REFERENCE TO THE RECIPE.

## 'LOVE MYSELF' BODY BUTTER

This body mousse will leave your skin super hydrated and nourished. Apricot oil will help it to penetrate quickly. I recommend using citrus scents for winter months and refreshing herbal scents for summer.

- 150 g shea butter
- 50 g coconut oil
- 50 g apricot oil
- 20 drops vitamin E
- 40 drops essential oil, as below depending on the season:
  Winter: 20 tangerine, 10 lemon and 10 petitgrain or grapefruit
  Summer: 30 lavender and 10 rosemary

## 'I LOVE YOU TOO' BODY BUTTER

Delicious body butter based on cocoa butter and chocolate, ideal for sharing. Fully edible.

- 125 g cocoa butter
- 125 g coconut oil
- 20 drops vitamin E
- 1 tablespoon pure cocoa powder
- 10 drops edible vanilla extract (optional)

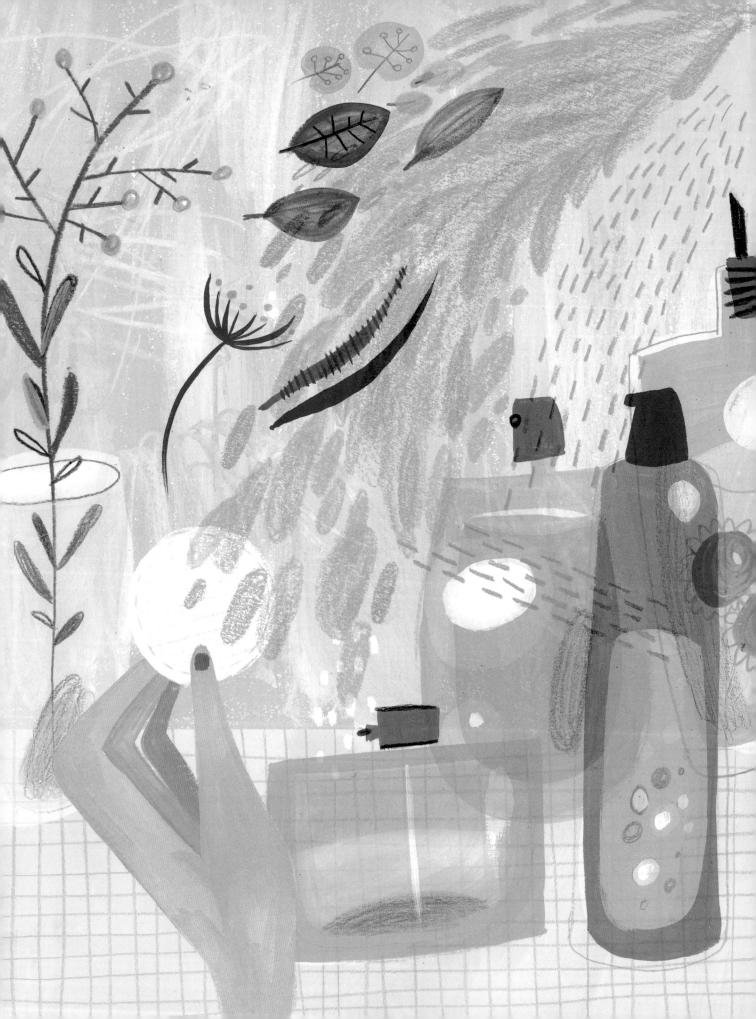

# hydrosols and floral watERS

We associate the concept of toning with a classic beauty ritual. Toners are usually used after removing make-up from the face, to close pores and to feel the fresh sensation of cleanliness. That's what it's all about.

In natural skin care, there are recipes for several types of preparations whose common element is water. The best way to do this is by infusion or boiling, which you can do at home, using plants that you are interested in and taking advantage of the active ingredients that dissolve in the water. An infusion can be a good tonic, hair rinse or watery base for a shampoo or soap. They are usually made with distilled water, as it is demineralised and has less possibility of contamination.

The waters that are all the rage in organic cosmetics are the floral ones, also called hydrosols or hydrolates (don't confuse them with infusions!). Hydrosols are the waters left over from the steam distillation process carried out on plants and flowers in order to extract their essential oil. Today they are used for medicinal, cosmetic and culinary uses, as they have water-soluble molecules similar to those of essential oils, although to a lesser degree. They can be used topically without a problem (unless you have an allergy to a particular oil). Rose, lavender, jasmine, witch-hazel, rosemary and chamomile are some of the most commonly used hydrosols in cosmetics. By themselves, they are very powerful, and they can be used to make facial and hair tonics, masks, creams, lotions and mouthwashes.

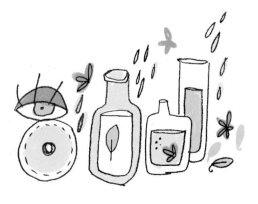

# INFUSIONS AND WATERS

Medicinal plant infusions can work perfectly as facial toners. There are different infusions for different skin types and ailments. Store them in the fridge, for no more than 3 days.

 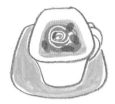 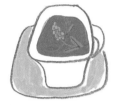 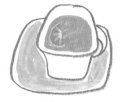

### CHAMOMILE AND MARIGOLD TONIC

Fantastic infusion for inflamed and irritated skin, dermatitis, etc..

- 1 small cup distilled water
- 15 g chamomile flowers
- 15 g marigold flowers

Heat the water and add the flowers when it begins to boil, then leave to sit for a while. Strain the infusion and, when it is cold, transfer it to a bottle and keep it in the fridge.

### TONIC OF ROSE PETALS

(for mature skin)

- 1 small cup distilled water
- 50 g rose petals of controlled origin (avoid florist ones as they are often treated with pesticides)

Boil the petals in the water over very low heat for a couple of minutes. Strain, let cool and transfer the liquid to a spray bottle and keep it in the fridge..

### MARIGOLD FLOWER AND LAVENDER TONIC

(for normal and combination skin)

- 1 small cup distilled water
- 15 g lavender petals
- 15 g marigold petals

Heat the water, then add the flowers when the water begins to boil. Turn off the heat and let sit for a while. Strain the infusion and, when it is cold, transfer it to a bottle and keep it in the fridge.

### GREEN TEA TONIC WITH LEMON JUICE

(anti-inflammatory, antioxidant, especially for oily and acne-prone skin)

- 1 small cup distilled water
- 10 g green tea
- 20 g chamomile flowers
- 1 splash of lemon juice

Boil the water, then add the tea and flowers and leave to infuse for 5 minutes. Strain and let cool. Add a squeeze of lemon and pour the infusion into a spray bottle. Keep it in the fridge.

### RICE WATER
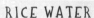

Rice water is based on the traditional rituals of Asian women, and is popular in K-beauty. Apply it with a cotton ball to the face and neck before going to bed.

- 300 ml distilled water
- 100 g organically grown rice

Rinse the rice a little and place it in a bowl. Add the water to cover it, then stir and let it rest for about 30 minutes. Strain, the rice water into a bottle and store in the fridge. There are some recipes that recommend letting the water ferment for a couple of days at room temperature before it is refrigerated.

### OAT WATER

This water, perfect for eczema and sensitive skin, will help reduce pimples and impurities, and calm irritated and sensitive skin. In a very clean saucepan place:

- 1 litre (34 fl oz) distilled water
- 25 g organically grown oats

Set the mixture on a very low heat, without letting it boil, for 5 to 10 minutes. Let it cool and strain it, reserving the liquid then transfer it to a spray bottle. Keep it in the fridge. It will last for about a week.

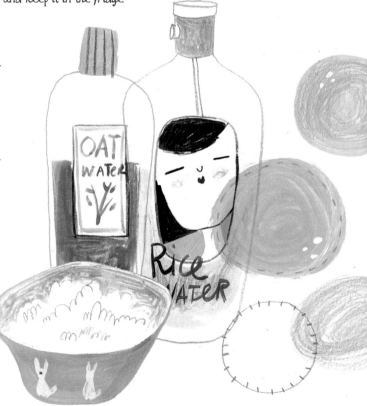

# HYDROSOLS AND SKIN TYPES

Hydrosols have properties that are similar to essential oils from the same plant but milder. They are ideal in organic skin care, since they work as tonics that can also be used as water bases for creams. There is no specific hydrosol for each type of skin. Use this table as a guide, as there are hydrosols compatible with all skin types.

| SKIN TYPE | NORMAL | DRY | OILY | MIXED | SENSITIVE | MATURE | ACNE-PRONE |
|---|---|---|---|---|---|---|---|
| HYDROSOL | lavender rose mint orange blossom green tea geranium | rose jasmine cornflower | witch-hazel lavender rosemary tea tree orange blossom thyme | lavender orange blossom witch-hazel mint geranium | chamomile lavender jasmine orange blossom rock rose | rose jasmine lemon balm rock rose green tea cornflower | witch-hazel thyme orange blossom tea tree rosemary rock rose mint |

## TWO-STEP MAKE-UP REMOVER FOR FACE AND EYES

If you are bothered by the feeling of using oils for removing make-up, here's a recipe that you'll love. It is fantastic for the hot months, since the hydrosol will provide a pleasant feeling of freshness.

In a pretty bottle, mix:

- 40 g of a hydrosol suitable for your skin
- 30 g castor oil
- 30 g jojoba oil
  (if you have dry skin, use almond or olive oil)
- 2 drops vitamin E

Shake the bottle before each application to homogenise the mixture.

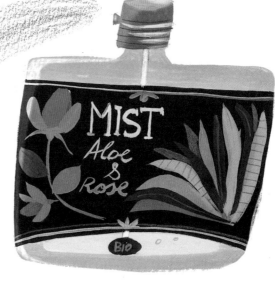

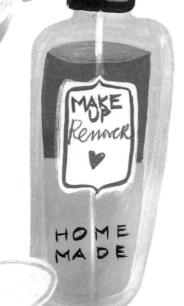

## ALOE VERA AND ROSE REFRESHING MIST

Use this spray on your face and body, or even in your hair. Fantastic to hydrate and freshen up after the office or travelling. Keep it in the fridge.

In a plastic spray bottle mix:

- 50 g aloe vera gel
- 50 g rose hydrosol
  (or mint is ideal for summer)
- a little distilled water to thin the mixture

Shake the bottle before each application to homogenise the mixture.

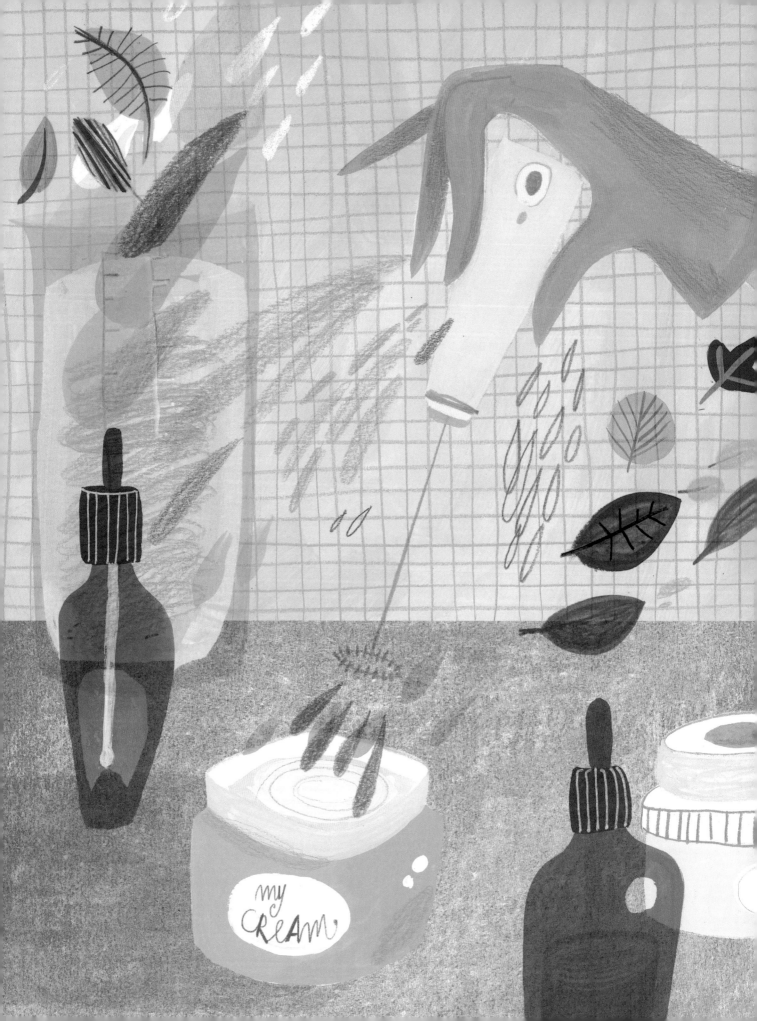

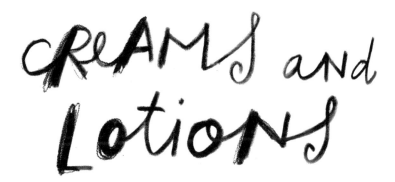

# CREAMS and LOTIONS

Testing textures, smells, combining ingredients ... Making creams is as pleasurable for me as mixing crayons and watercolours in my drawings. Making your own creams opens up a world of recipes and endless combinations. If you are interested in the subject, I suggest you try to get as much information about the ingredients and their benefits as possible to help you understand how to use them correctly.

In previous chapters, we have covered butters, oils and floral waters. Now it is time to combine them. A cream is an emulsion where two liquids that are separate in their natural state, such as oil and water, are mixed together. This is where the term emulsifier comes from: it is an essential ingredient that stabilises the mixture and prevents the two ingredients from separating. There are plenty of certified organic emulsifiers (for example, made from olive, wheat or soy) that you can buy in specialised stores or online. Beeswax and lecithin are also emulsifiers.

Adding water to the mixtures opens the doors to the possibility of fungi and bacteria making an appearance. Although essential oils have antifungal and antibacterial powers, sometimes that's not enough. There are preservatives on the market (Xaromix, Geogard, Leucidal, Rokonsal, etc.) that have safety certifications and are free of parabens and can extend the life of a cream for up to 4 months. Personally, I recommend making small batches and using them for a couple of months at most. If you store the cream in an airtight container and use a plastic spoon (which you wash after each application) to take it out, you will avoid putting your fingers in the cream, which will also protect it from possible contamination.

During the hotter months, store creams in the fridge. This will extend their life and you will appreciate the fresh sensation when applying them.

You will need, in addition to the equipment you have used so far, a small battery-powered hand mixer (to whip cocktails or creams) and test strips for measuring pH. It is important that creams respect the natural pH level of the acid mantle, which is the slightly acidic film on the surface of our skin.

If you're just starting out, don't forget to do a small patch test in the crease of your elbow before applying a product to your face. You may be sensitive or allergic to some component. Just because the ingredients come from natural sources does not mean that they can't cause a reaction.

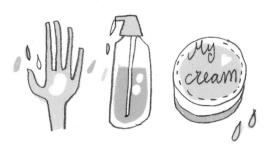

# BASIC EMULSION

Making an emulsion with water and oil is easy, but you must follow a series of steps as well as some basic rules. Soon you'll see that it is very easy and fun! Before starting, take a good look at the diagrams on these pages and try to understand the entire production process. Clean and disinfect all containers (don't forget the end of the mixer and the scales) and wipe surfaces with alcohol. Wear gloves or wash your hands well with hot water.

## MATERIALS

- 2 heat-resistant containers
- thermometer
- weighing scales
- small blender or stick mixer
- pH measuring strips
- pot for the bain-marie
- ice bowl to cool the mixture

WHEN MAKING A CREAM OR EMULSION, YOU MUST TAKE INTO ACCOUNT THREE DIFFERENT PHASES, DEPENDING ON THE TYPE OF INGREDIENTS YOU ARE USING:

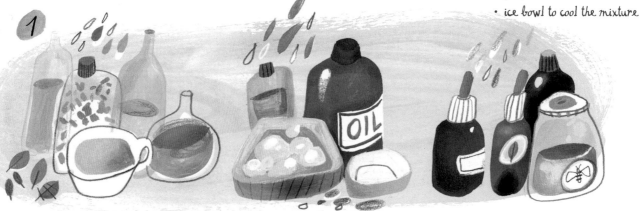

### HYDROSOLS (PHASE A)

In this phase we group the ingredients that contain water (distilled water, hydrosol, glycerine, infusion, etc.).

### OILS (PHASE B)

In this phase we group all the fatty ingredients (oils, butters, waxes, etc.).

### ADDITIVES (PHASE C)

In this phase we add additives that should not be exposed to high temperatures at the end of the preparation (essential oils, vitamin E, honey, preservatives, etc.).

YOU NEED TO USE A THERMOMETER TO CONTROL THE TEMPERATURES OF EACH CONTAINER. BOTH MUST REACH 70°C (158°F) AT THE SAME TIME. IF ONE HEATS UP BEFORE THE OTHER, TAKE IT OUT OF THE POT WHILE YOU WAIT FOR THE TEMPERATURE OF THE OTHER TO RISE. IF IT GETS TOO COLD, PUT IT BACK IN.

YOU MUST BE VERY ATTENTIVE, AS THIS STEP IS IMPORTANT. WHEN THEY ARE BOTH AT THE CORRECT TEMPERATURE, REMOVE THEM FROM THE HEAT.

2. USE TWO CONTAINERS: ONE FOR THE HYDROSOLS (PHASE A) AND THE OTHER FOR THE OILS (PHASE B).

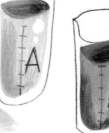

3. ONCE YOU HAVE WEIGHED THE INGREDIENTS FOR EACH PHASE, PUT THEM IN THEIR RESPECTIVE CONTAINERS AND PUT THEM IN THE BAIN-MARIE.

MIX WITH A STIRRER WHILE THEY HEAT. REMEMBER THE WATER IN THE POT SHOULD NEVER BOIL.

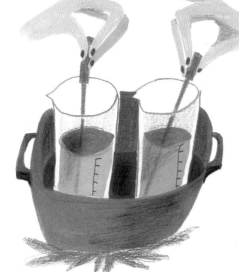

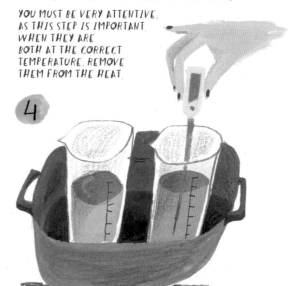

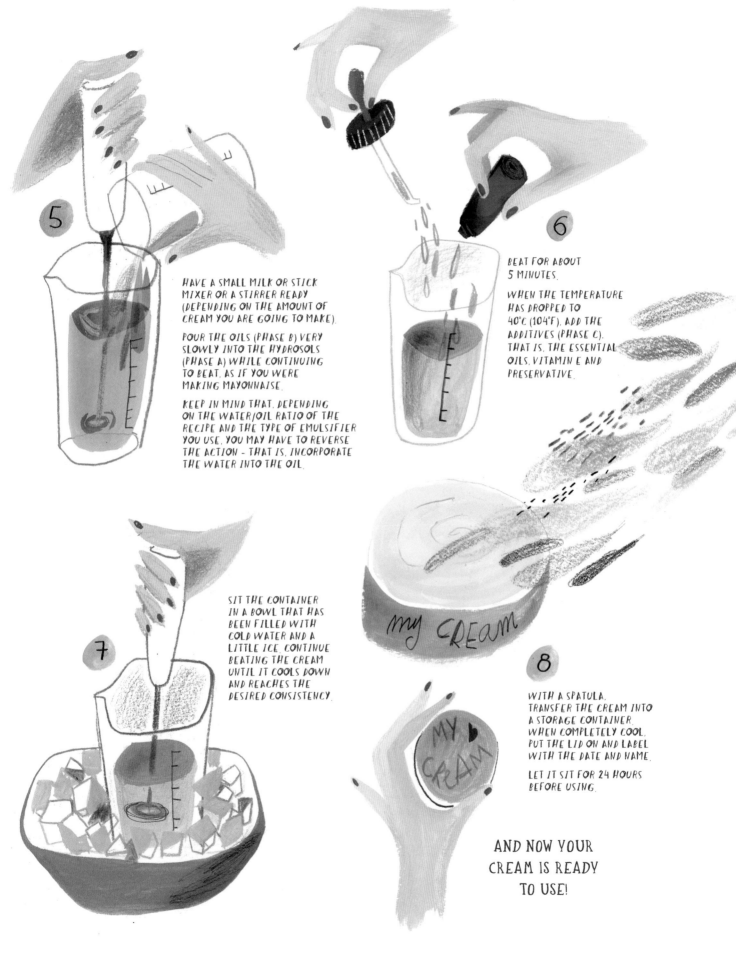

**5**

HAVE A SMALL MILK OR STICK MIXER OR A STIRRER READY (DEPENDING ON THE AMOUNT OF CREAM YOU ARE GOING TO MAKE).

POUR THE OILS (PHASE B) VERY SLOWLY INTO THE HYDROSOLS (PHASE A) WHILE CONTINUING TO BEAT, AS IF YOU WERE MAKING MAYONNAISE.

KEEP IN MIND THAT, DEPENDING ON THE WATER/OIL RATIO OF THE RECIPE AND THE TYPE OF EMULSIFIER YOU USE, YOU MAY HAVE TO REVERSE THE ACTION - THAT IS, INCORPORATE THE WATER INTO THE OIL.

**6**

BEAT FOR ABOUT 5 MINUTES.

WHEN THE TEMPERATURE HAS DROPPED TO 40°C (104°F), ADD THE ADDITIVES (PHASE C), THAT IS, THE ESSENTIAL OILS, VITAMIN E AND PRESERVATIVE.

**7**

SIT THE CONTAINER IN A BOWL THAT HAS BEEN FILLED WITH COLD WATER AND A LITTLE ICE. CONTINUE BEATING THE CREAM UNTIL IT COOLS DOWN AND REACHES THE DESIRED CONSISTENCY.

*my* CREAM

**8**

WITH A SPATULA, TRANSFER THE CREAM INTO A STORAGE CONTAINER. WHEN COMPLETELY COOL, PUT THE LID ON AND LABEL WITH THE DATE AND NAME.

LET IT SIT FOR 24 HOURS BEFORE USING.

MY CREAM

AND NOW YOUR CREAM IS READY TO USE!

# CREAMS

## BASIC CLASSIC COLD CREAM

Cold cream is one of the oldest known creams, attributed to Galen, an historical Greek doctor. It is moisturising, soothing and nourishing. It is one of my favourite creams because of its wonderful properties and the simplicity of its formula and preparation. Make sure the ingredients are of the highest quality. This recipe has lasted through time and it seems that we are always rediscovering it. Do not miss it!

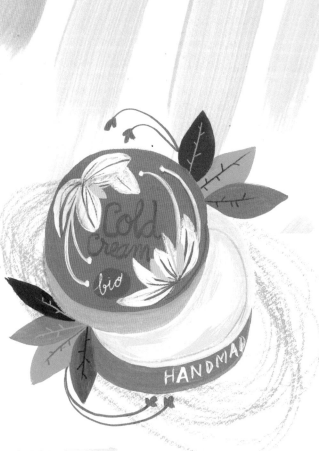

### HYDROSOL (PHASE A)
- 25 g rose hydrosol

### OILS (PHASE B)
- 22 g olive or almond oil
- 2.5 g beeswax

### ADDITIVES (PHASE C)
- 5 drops vitamin E
- 6 drops damask rose essential oil
- 3 drops preservative (check the manufacturer's recommended proportions)

WEIGH THE INGREDIENTS AND PLACE THEM IN THEIR CONTAINERS, BASED ON WHAT PHASE THEY ARE IN.

HEAT THE OILS (PHASE B) IN THE BAIN-MARIE UNTIL THE WAX IS COMPLETELY MELTED.

THE HYDROSOL (PHASE A) SHOULD SIMPLY BE WARMED, YOU CAN HEAT IT IN THE BAIN-MARIE FOR 1 MINUTE.

POUR THE HYDROSOL INTO THE OILS VERY SLOWLY, WHILE YOU MIX WITH THE MIXER, YOU MUST LET THE CREAM COOL WHILE CONTINUING TO MIX.

ADD THE ADDITIVES (PHASE C) AND CONTINUE BEATING UNTIL YOU GET A SMOOTH, THICK CREAM.

## SOOTHING CLEANSING CREAM

If you are not used to oil-based cleansing and prefer a classic cleansing cream, this is a recipe that, in addition to cleansing and removing make-up, will soothe your skin, leaving it refreshed. It's made with aloe, macerated flower oil, coconut and castor oil. Store in an air-tight bottle. Apply it with your fingers and remove it with cotton discs soaked with a hydrosol that suits your skin.

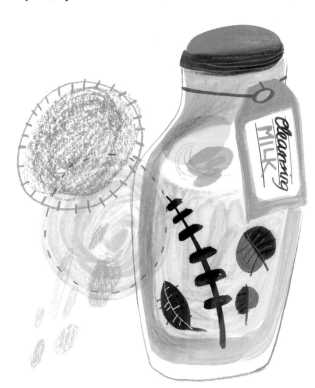

### HYDROSOLS (PHASE A)
- 18 g chamomile hydrosol
- 10 g aloe vera gel
- 10 drops vegetable glycerine

### OILS (PHASE B)
- 6 g lavender and chamomile macerated oil
- 6 g coconut oil
- 4 g castor oil
- 2 g beeswax
- 1.5 g olive-derived emulsifier

### ADDITIVES (PHASE C)
- 5 drops vitamin E
- 6 drops lavender essential oil
- 3 drops preservative (check the manufacturer's recommended proportions)

(FOLLOW THE STEP-BY-STEP INSTRUCTIONS ON PAGES 104-105)

WEIGH THE INGREDIENTS AND PLACE THEM IN THEIR CONTAINERS, BASED ON WHAT PHASE THEY ARE.

PLACE THEM IN THE BAIN-MARIE AND REMOVE THEM WHEN THEY REACH 70°C (158°F).

SLOWLY POUR THE OILS INTO THE HYDROSOLS WHILE BEATING CONTINUOUSLY. WHEN THE TEMPERATURE LOWERS, INTRODUCE THE ADDITIVES AND MEASURE THE PH.

STAND THE CONTAINER IN A BOWL WITH COLD WATER AND ICE TO COOL.

LET STAND, COVER, THEN LABEL WITH NAME AND DATE.

## CREAM FOR MATURE SKIN

This cream has a creamy texture because it has a high level of fat. Fantastic for dry, mature skin or as a night cream. Avocado oil and rosehip oil are nourishing and repairing. The wheatgerm oil adds antioxidants, so there is no need to add vitamin E. The wonderful essential oils of frankincense and ylang ylang will restore damaged skin and relax fine lines.

### HYDROSOLS (PHASE A)
- 28 g rose hydrosol
- 10 drops vegetable glycerine

### OILS (PHASE B)
- 6 g shea butter
- 5 g avocado oil
- 4 g rosehip oil
- 2 g wheatgerm oil
- 2 g virgin beeswax
- 1.5 g olive-derived emulsifier

### ADDITIVES (PHASE C)
- 3 drops frankincense essential oil
- 3 drops ylang ylang essential oil
- 3 drops preservative (check the manufacturer's recommended proportions)

## CREAM FOR NORMAL SKIN

This is a fairly light cream, with almond oil and coconut oil to nourish your skin and provide elasticity. Aloe vera and lavender hydrosol will compensate for the fats and add lightness and freshness to the preparation. For daily use.

### HYDROSOLS (PHASE A)
- 22 g lavender hydrosol
- 8 g aloe vera gel

### OILS (PHASE B)
- 6 g shea butter
- 6 g almond oil
- 4 g coconut oil
- 2 g virgin beeswax
- 1,5 g olive-derived emulsifier

### ADDITIVES (PHASE C)
- 4 drops vitamin E
- 4 drops lavender essential oil
- 2 drops geranium essential oil
- 3 drops preservative (check the manufacturer's recommended proportions)

## LOTION FOR OILY SKIN

A light lotion for oily skin and fantastic for summer. Witch-hazel is a powerful astringent and jojoba and grapeseed oils are very quickly absorbed. If you have a tendency to acne, substitute castor oil for jojoba oil. If your skin has a tendency to shine, add half a teaspoon of cornflour (cornstarch).

### HYDROSOLS (PHASE A)
- 35 g witch-hazel hydrosol
- 15 g aloe vera gel
- 10 drops vegetable glycerine

### OILS (PHASE B)
- 7 g jojoba oil (or castor oil)
- 4 g grapeseed oil
- 3 g olive-derived emulsifier

### ADDITIVES (PHASE C)
- 4 drops vitamin E
- 3 drops lavender essential oil
- 3 drops tea tree essential oil
- 3 drops preservative (check the manufacturer's recommended proportions)

Follow the steps on pages 104 and 105 to make these creams. In the first two recipes, add the minimum amount of emulsifier, since beeswax also acts as an emulsifier.

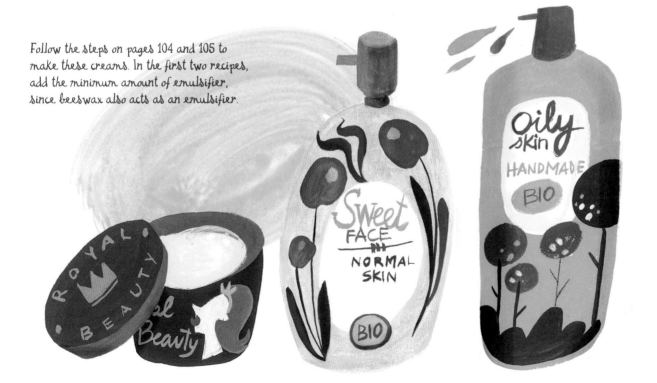

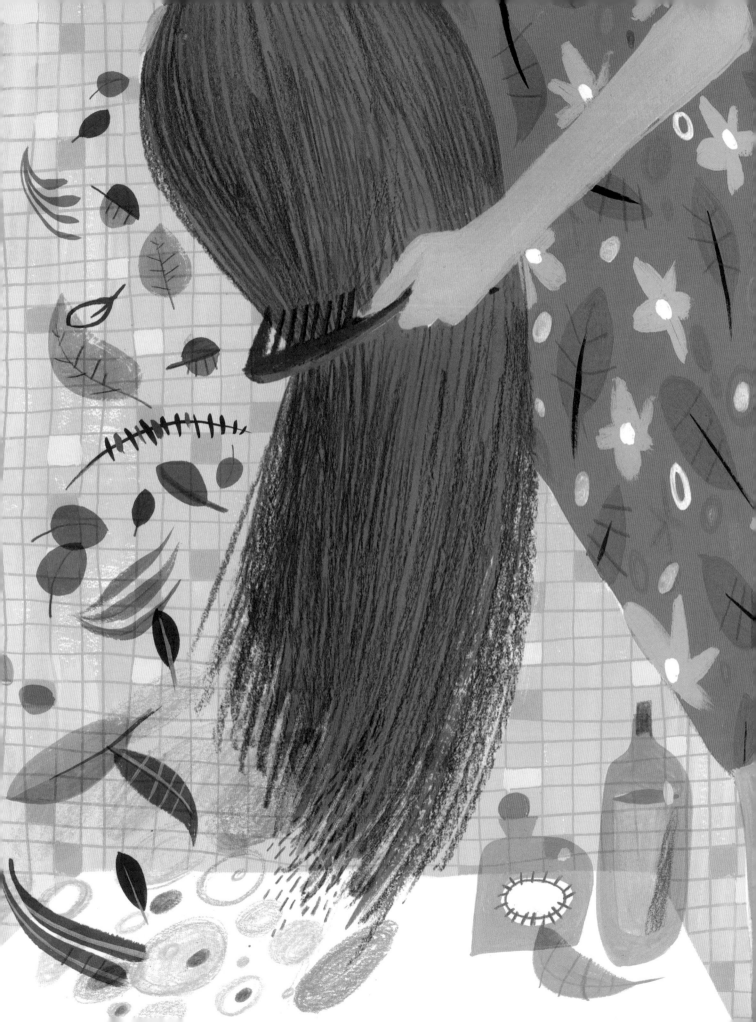

# hAiR cARe

Who wouldn't want thick, shiny hair flowing down their shoulders? Hair has a lot to do with our image and we are often unhappy with it.

It is a part of our body that suffers the most chemical assaults: silicons, sulphates, parabens and unclassifiable fragrances contained in shampoos and masks, ammonia and solvents in dyes and straightening treatments ... the list goes on. Hair chemistry is very complex and intense, but offers the magic of brightness, density and colour changes almost instantly. It's possible that if you are changing from store-bought hair-care products to homemade ones, you may feel some frustration with the initial results.

Making an organic shampoo with a gel consistency means entering the world of surfactants (emulsifiers that generate foam with cleansing capabilities). Getting to know them and combining them to get good results is not an easy task. In natural cosmetics, natural-origin surfactants are used, such as coco betaine, coco glucoside and decyl glucoside, which, together with edible gelling agents (xanthan gum or guar gum), vegetable oils, infusions and hydrosols, make shampoos that you can adapt to target many different hair needs.

If you are interested in hair cosmetics, there are specific publications and workshops that can help you make your own products, but to begin with, I advise you to experiment with neutral bases, such as certified organic shampoo or liquid Castile soap, to which you can add vegetable oils, essential oils or infusions, easily customising them according to your tastes.

During perimenopause, I began to develop serious intolerances to chemical hair dyes, as well as drastic hair loss. And while I love grey hair, I didn't feel ready to keep it. Dyeing my hair myself with henna has been one of the greatest successes that I have adopted from the world of natural cosmetics, not only for having freed myself from chemical dyes, but also for the joy of a new level of strong, healthy hair.

In Ayurvedic cosmetics, which concentrate on a holistic approach, there are plants that offer fantastic results when used for hair care. They are sold in powder form, for example shikakai, neem and amla powder, and they are mixed with water or an infusion, then applied as a hair mask. Other types of natural hair treatments are rinses, especially those made with plants like rosemary, nettle, horsetail, soapwort and burdock, or macerated dyes you can make with them.

Last, but not least, don't forget to use a natural bristle brush and massage your scalp well.

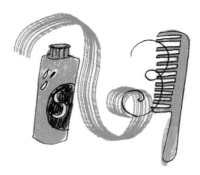

# STEP-BY-STEP: HENNA DYE

Henna comes from a shrub (*Lawsonia inermis*) that grows in arid climates. Its leaves, since ancient times, have been dried and powdered to make hair dye and used for skin tattoos. A paste made from the powder will dye and strengthen your hair. The tone is rather reddish, but when mixed with other herbs, such as indigo (which is black in colour), you can make other colours. Using the same method, you can apply cassia, also known as neutral henna, which has the same benefits as henna, adding strength and shine, but has very little dye in it. It's also good for preventing lice. Or you can use amla (on its own or combined with henna), an Ayurvedic plant that strengthens the hair and stimulates growth.

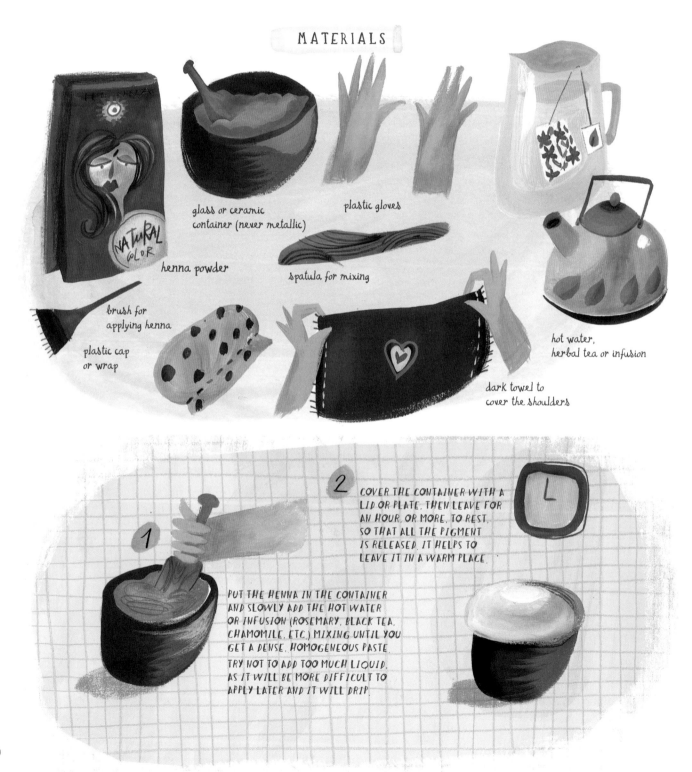

MATERIALS

henna powder

glass or ceramic
container (never metallic)

plastic gloves

brush for
applying henna

plastic cap
or wrap

spatula for mixing

dark towel to
cover the shoulders

hot water,
herbal tea or infusion

1 — PUT THE HENNA IN THE CONTAINER AND SLOWLY ADD THE HOT WATER OR INFUSION (ROSEMARY, BLACK TEA, CHAMOMILE, ETC.) MIXING UNTIL YOU GET A DENSE, HOMOGENEOUS PASTE. TRY NOT TO ADD TOO MUCH LIQUID, AS IT WILL BE MORE DIFFICULT TO APPLY LATER AND IT WILL DRIP.

2 — COVER THE CONTAINER WITH A LID OR PLATE, THEN LEAVE FOR AN HOUR, OR MORE, TO REST, SO THAT ALL THE PIGMENT IS RELEASED. IT HELPS TO LEAVE IT IN A WARM PLACE.

MEANWHILE, PROTECT THE AREA
WHERE YOU ARE GOING TO WORK WITH
NEWSPAPERS OR PLASTIC. REMEMBER THAT
YOU MUST HAVE CLEAN AND DRY HAIR.

APPLY A BALM OR SOME OLD SUNSCREEN TO
THE ROOTS OF THE HAIR, EARS, AND NAPE
OF THE NECK, AND PUT ON OLD CLOTHES.

BY NOW THE HENNA WILL BE A DARK BROWN
COLOUR. PUT ON YOUR GLOVES, STAND IN FRONT
OF A MIRROR AND START APPLYING.

START WITH THE BACK OF THE HEAD, SECTION BY
SECTION, USING THE DYE BRUSH, MAKING SURE
THAT THE ROOTS ARE WELL SATURATED WITH THE
PASTE. APPLY THE REST WITH YOUR HANDS AND AT
THE END MASSAGE WELL INTO YOUR SCALP.

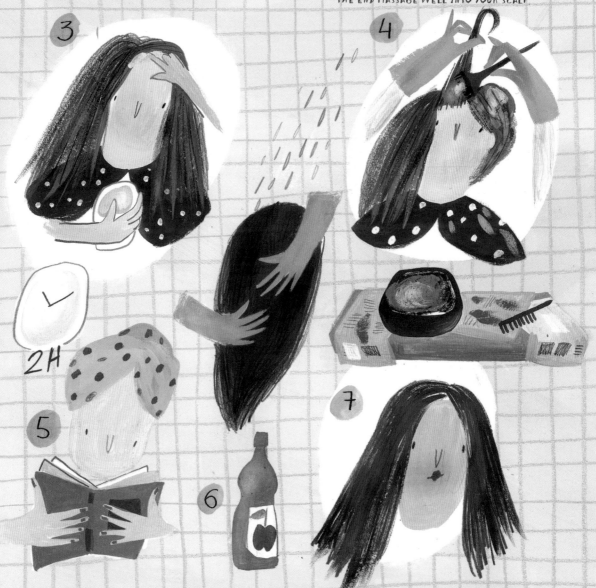

WRAP YOUR HEAD WITH PLASTIC WRAP OR
PUT ON A PLASTIC CAP. COVER WITH A TOWEL
SO THE HENNA STAYS MOIST AND WARM.

LEAVE FOR A MINIMUM OF 2 OR 3 HOURS. (SOME PEOPLE
LEAVE IT IN ALL NIGHT). ORGANISE THAT TIME SO YOU
DON'T HAVE TO LEAVE HOME. I USE THIS TIME TO MAKE
SOAPS AND COSMETICS. REMEMBER TO CLEAN THE GLOVES,
AS YOU WILL NEED THEM TO REMOVE THE HENNA.

WHEN THE TIME IS UP, RINSE OFF THE HENNA,
UNTIL THE WATER COMES OUT CLEAR.

MAKE AN APPLE CIDER VINEGAR RINSE (1 PART VINEGAR TO
3 PARTS WATER), AND USE THAT AS THE FINAL RINSE TO CLOSE
THE CUTICLES. IF THE ENDS ARE VERY DRY, USE A LITTLE
COCONUT OIL TO UNTANGLE THEM. DRY IN THE SUN IF YOU CAN.
WAIT A COUPLE OF DAYS BEFORE SHAMPOOING YOUR HAIR.
REMEMBER TO USE DARK TOWELS FOR THE NEXT FEW DAYS,
AS YOU WILL LOSE COLOUR IN THE FIRST FEW WASHES.

# A LA CARTE SHAMPOOS

By using the famous Castile soap as a base and adding various ingredients, we can adapt recipes to suit different types of hair. The amounts below are indicative, since Castile soap can be diluted by up to one-third. A system of trial and error works best to find the result that you like the most. Make small batches, rounding up or down to suit. For ease, mix everything in a plastic bottle with a dispenser. Remember that an acid rinse (made with vinegar or lemon) at the end of the wash will help balance pH levels.
Here are some recipes for different types of hair:

### MOISTURISING

- 100 g liquid Castile soap
- 50 g aloe vera
- 50 g lavender infusion
- 4 g almond oil
- 1 teaspoon xanthan gum (to thicken)
- 6 drops ylang ylang essential oil
- 6 drops lavender essential oil

### FOR OILY HAIR

- 100 g liquid Castile soap
- 100 g nettle infusion
- 2 g jojoba oil
- 1 teaspoon kaolin (white clay)
- 1 teaspoon xanthan gum (to thicken)
- 8 drops lemon essential oil
- 4 drops tea tree essential oil

### FOR FINE HAIR

- 100 g liquid Castile soap
- 100 g infusion of marigold and chamomile or oat water*
- 3 g almond oil
- 1 teaspoon xanthan gum (to thicken)
- 4 drops lavender essential oil
- 4 drops chamomile essential oil

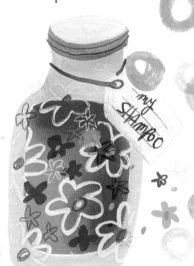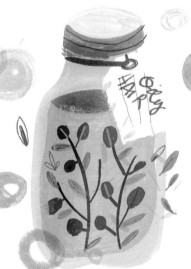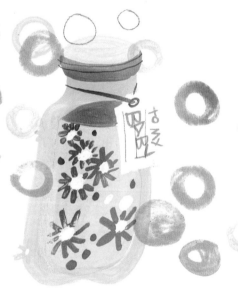

*The oat water can be made by leaving 2 tablespoons of colloidal oatmeal to soak in 200 g of distilled water. Place over a low heat for about 10 minutes to release the mucilage but don't allow it to boil. Blend, then pass through a coarse sieve.

### DRY SHAMPOO

Want to last longer between washes? Are you in a period of hormonal changes and find you have a greasy scalp? This recipe can help. Mix the ingredients carefully and add the essential oil at the last moment. You can recycle a clean spice container to store it. Apply the mixture to the roots, leave for a few minutes then brush well.

- 20 g cornflour (cornstarch) or arrowroot
- 20 g rice flour
- 10 g baking soda
- 6 drops lavender essential oil

### ROSEMARY AND NETTLE HAIR TONIC

This hair tonic is fantastic for strengthening hair and stopping hair loss. Put the herbs and vodka in a glass jar. Let the preparation macerate for approximately 20 days in a dark place. Shake the jar frequently. Strain it and store it in a dark glass bottle. Before washing your hair, give yourself a good scalp massage with this mixture.

- 1 litre (34 fl oz) vodka
- 200 g rosemary
- 100 g nettle leaves
- 10 drops rosemary essential oil (optional)

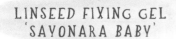

## LINSEED FIXING GEL 'SAYONARA BABY'

This fixing gel, as well as creating beautiful waves and helping to style your hair, has lots of benefits due to the omega-3 fatty acids that provide your hair with strength and nutrients. You can also use it as a softener after washing, adding a squeeze of lemon to close the cuticles. Try it - you will be pleasantly surprised!

Bring the water and seeds to the boil. When it begins to thicken (keeping in mind that when it cools it thickens more) remove it from the heat and strain through a coarse sieve, so that all the viscous fluid passes through. Leave to cool, then stir through the remaining ingredients. Store it in the fridge. As always when using water, add a few drops of preservative

- 100 g distilled water
- 25 g linseeds (flax seeds)
- a squeeze of lemon juice
- 1 g vegetable glycerine (optional)
- 10 drops preservative (check the manufacturer's recommended proportions)
- 10 drops essential oil of your choice

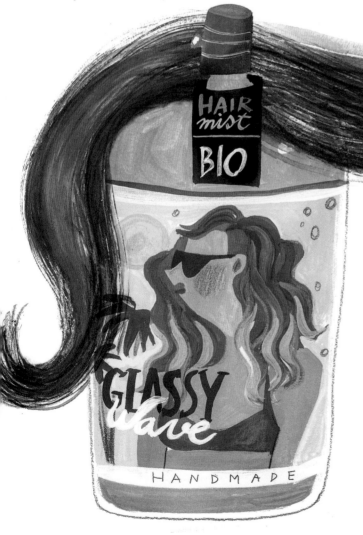

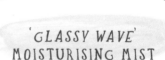

## 'GLASSY WAVE' MOISTURISING MIST

Do you want a beach vibe, like a surfer's waves? This fantastic spray will set your curls and provide hydration, as well as a lovely holiday feeling. Gently heat the distilled water and add all the ingredients, letting them sit until they are completely dissolved. Put them in a plastic spray bottle and let cool. Shake well before use

- 150 g sea or distilled water
- 15 g aloe vera
- 10 g Epsom salts
- 5 g white sugar
- 5 g liquid coconut or jojoba oil
- 2 g vegetable glycerine (optional)
- 2 drops ylang ylang essential oil

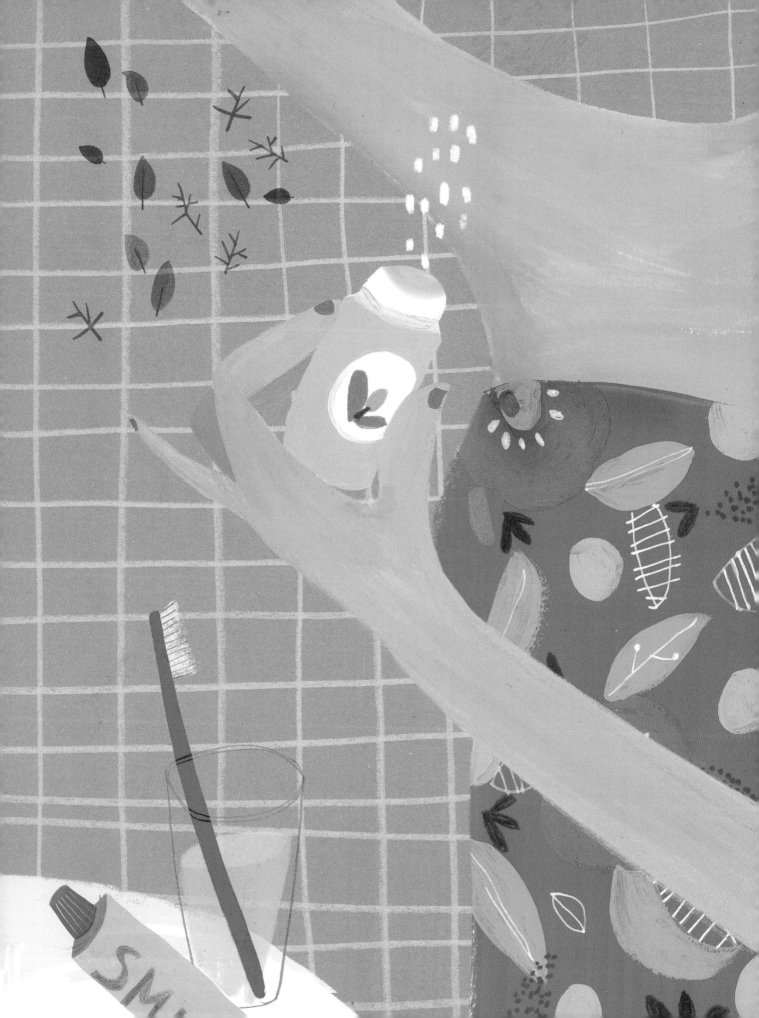

# dEoDoRaNts aNd ORal cARe

There are many controversies on the subject of deodorants – hundreds of papers have been written on their dangerous ingredients and their relationship to serious diseases. Beyond the aesthetic component, sweat and bad body odour can be real problems for many women, especially during times of hormonal changes or stress.

It's a complex issue. Sweating and bad body odour can be linked to lots of factors that may need to be checked by a doctor or dietitian. Sweat is a reflection of what is happening inside us and there are many causes: hormonal changes, stress and medications, to name a few.

In natural cosmetics, there are no really effective solutions for the most severe cases. There are many antiperspirant products that eradicate sweat by clogging the sweat glands, but studies show that they can have negative long-term health consequences. Aluminium and parabens, as well as certain fragrances, are common components in conventional deodorants and generate a lot of controversy. Many people believe that they are potentially dangerous and, as sometimes is the case, consumers don't know the full truth.

Ingredients such as bicarbonate, kaolin, cornflour (cornstarch) and certain essential oils have properties that counteract the effects of sweat. Although their effectiveness is relative compared to conventional deodorants, they can work very well in many cases. Personally, I am happy with them (although sometimes I have to apply them several times a day). I can only advise you to try. They are not expensive and they are harmless.

The same narrative applies to toothpastes and mouthwashes, where the supposed dangerous potential of some of their components is multiplied, as they are in contact with the mucous membranes and open wounds in the mouth. But, like sweat, teeth are also a reflection of our internal state, as well as our eating and hygiene habits.

There is some research that proves the effectiveness of coconut oil to fight some bacteria that accumulate in the mouth and teeth. Combined with baking soda and some choice essential oils, such as mint, clove, thyme and chamomile, they can be a good alternative if you don't have any serious problems or concerns. Do you dare to try?

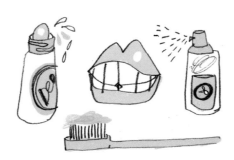

# DEODORANTS

In natural cosmetics, there are a number of ingredients recommended for making deodorants and which are common to most recipes: coconut oil, for its antibacterial and anti-inflammatory capacity; cornflour (cornstarch) or arrowroot, which absorb moisture and protect you from irritations; bicarbonate to neutralise the bacteria that cause bad body odour; and tea tree essential oil, which is a powerful disinfectant. In addition, witch-hazel and sage hydrosols are suitable for making liquid deodorants, as is aloe vera, which softens and refreshes.

## STICK DEODORANT

To make this deodorant you need an empty stick container. You can recycle one you've got at home, or buy an empty container. You can add eucalyptus, rosemary, sage or lemon essential oils. Melt the cocoa butter and coconut oil in a heatproof container over a bain-marie. Remove from the heat and, when cooled, add the cornflour, baking soda and essential oils. Mix well and pour into the container. Modify the formula to suit the temperature of your home.

- 15 g coconut oil
- 30 g coconut oil
- 30 g cornflour (cornstarch)
- 15 g baking soda
- 10 drops essential oil of your choice

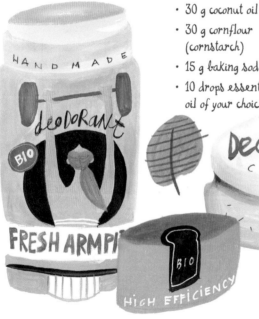

## ROLL-ON DEODORANT

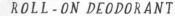

Mix the aloe vera gel and hydrosol. Add the baking soda and essential oils. You can recycle a used deodorant container - remove the ball, then put it back in place when filled.

- 30 g aloe vera gel
- 10 g sage hydrosol
- 5 g baking soda
- 4 drops essential oil (lemon, sage or lavender)

## CREAM DEODORANT

I package this deodorant in refillable plastic tubes when the mixture is still lukewarm, so that I can apply it without sticking my fingers into the jar and it's easy to carry. Modify the amount of coconut oil depending on your preferred texture. If you want it thinner, use liquid coconut oil, which doesn't harden. Melt the coconut oil in a water bath and add the remaining ingredients.

- 80 g coconut oil
- 30 g cornflour (cornstarch)
- 30 g baking soda
- 6 drops tea tree essential oil
- 3 drops sage or lavender essential oil

## SPRAY DEODORANT

I carry this deodorant with me to counteract the effects of sweat during a busy day. It refreshes and cleans. Vinegar neutralises odours and regulates the pH.

In a spray bottle mix:

- 20 g witch-hazel, sage or lavender hydrosol
- 20 g apple cider vinegar (if you don't like the smell, use 5 g)
- 5 g vodka (optional - don't add if you have easily irritated armpits)
- 10 drops vegetable glycerine
- 4 drops lemon essential oil
- 4 drops lavender essential oil

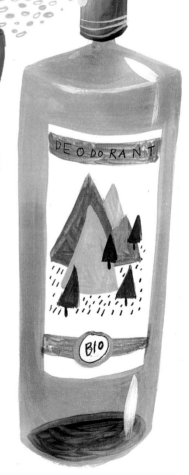

# ORAL CARE

There are alternatives to conventional products for oral care. In addition to oil pulling (which has been all the rage lately), you can make pastes and powders, using kaolin as a base and adding a little baking soda. By adding essential oils such as mint, rosemary or sage and a touch of stevia, you can make very pleasant flavours.

### OIL PULLING

Oil pulling is an Ayurvedic practice that consists of cleaning your mouth with oil to rid it of toxins and bacteria and promote stronger and healthier gums. When you get up, clean your tongue and rinse your mouth with water. Then take a tablespoon of coconut oil and slowly move it to all corners of your mouth as if you were rinsing. After 10 or 20 minutes, spit out the oil and rinse your mouth with warm water. Then brush your teeth as usual.

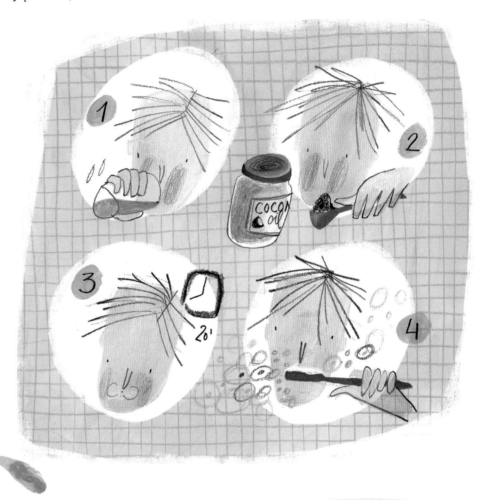

### KAOLIN AND MINT PASTE

This paste tastes fantastic and works really well. Melt the coconut oil then add the rest of the ingredients. Mix then pour the paste into a recyclable plastic jar or tube.

- 20 g coconut oil
- 5 g baking soda
- 8 g Kaolin (white clay)
- 2 drops mint essential oil
- pinch of stevia powder (optional)
- pinch of sea salt

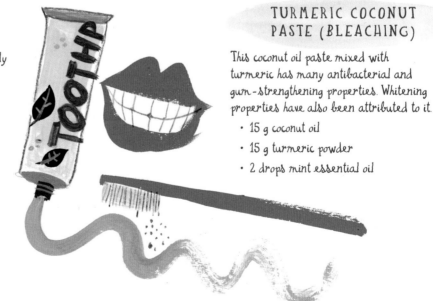

### TURMERIC COCONUT PASTE (BLEACHING)

This coconut oil paste mixed with turmeric has many antibacterial and gum-strengthening properties. Whitening properties have also been attributed to it.

- 15 g coconut oil
- 15 g turmeric powder
- 2 drops mint essential oil

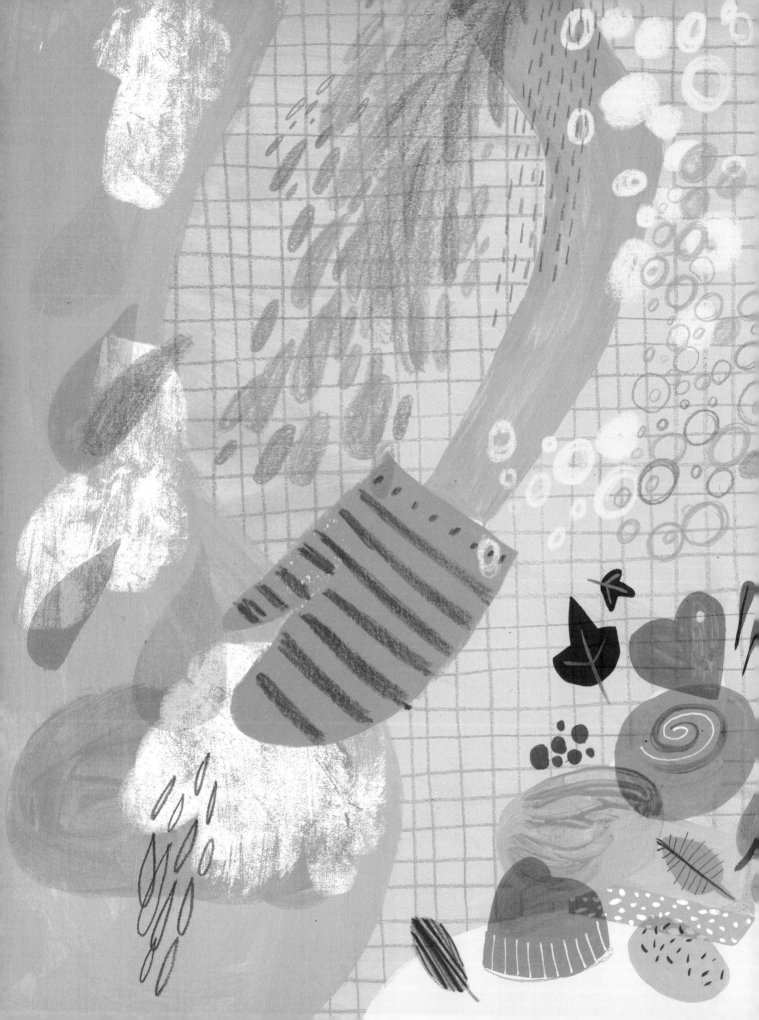

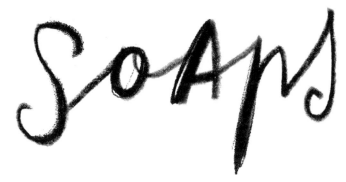

# Soaps

Available in infinite shapes, colours and smells, soaps unleash passions. The magic that occurs when we wet a bar and that creamy foam appears between our fingers has endured throughout the centuries. Although the Sumerians, Egyptians and Greeks already used soapy products, it was the Romans who dedicated themselves to making soap by hand. From its development comes the famous Castile soap and, later, Marseille soap. Let's not forget that the evolution of soap is linked to that of hygiene and health.

Soap is created by a chemical reaction between a fatty acid (oil or fat) and an alkali commonly known as caustic soda (sodium or potassium hydroxide). We call this process saponification – the transformation of a greasy substance into a product that makes stains and dirt dissolve in water.

Making homemade soap may seem fashionable, but in many countries it is a family tradition, like making jam or brandy. My family and I have been showering and washing our hands with soaps we make at home for years. Our soaps are made with freshly pressed oils that we buy in rural areas that have an abundance of olive and hazelnut trees. They are fat-rich soaps that hydrate and take care of our skin perfectly. I usually make them while I am dying my hair with henna (see page 110). I make a couple in long moulds and a series of individual soaps to which I add flower petals, plant-macerated oils or an exfoliator such as oatmeal or chia seeds. It's always exciting to prepare them then enjoy the result.

My advice is to try it, but be aware that making soaps can be very dangerous, especially if there are children or pets in your house. You have to handle caustic soda, which is a highly corrosive product that you must always keep under tight control. It can cause severe burns to the skin and eyes and is toxic if inhaled. You should only make soap in a well-ventilated space and wear gloves, a mask, goggles and old clothes to protect against any possible splashes. If you can work safely, then try them! I've included diagrams and a recipe on the following pages, but my advice is to make them first with someone who has experience, or attend a face-to-face workshop.

If this sounds too hard, there is a very safe and fun alternative – you can make 'melt and pour' glycerine soaps. All that's needed is to buy a glycerine soap base then melt it and pour it into moulds. Add whatever essential oils, clays, dried flowers or exfoliating ingredients you desire. Make sure these base ingredients are of a certified organic origin, and not of industrial origin with synthetic additives. There is a large market for attractive, colourful handmade soaps, which often unfortunately don't contain quality ingredients in the soap itself.

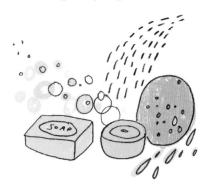

# CASTILE SOAP

Castile soap is one of the simplest and oldest known soaps. Unlike other soaps that are made with animal fats, this is made with olive oil, hence its wonderful properties. It doesn't foam much, but it is very moisturising and suitable for all skin types. Do you dare?

## PRECAUTIONS

- DO NOT MAKE SOAP IF THERE ARE CHILDREN, PETS OR PEOPLE COMING AND GOING IN YOUR HOUSE. YOU MUST BE RELAXED AND CALM. LOOK AT THE ILLUSTRATIONS DETAILING THE ENTIRE PROCESS SO YOU CAN SEE WHAT IT CONSISTS OF, FROM START TO FINISH, AND PROCEED AT YOUR OWN RISK. I STRONGLY RECOMMEND YOU FIRST MAKE IT WITH AN EXPERIENCED PERSON OR DO A PRACTICAL WORKSHOP.
- PROTECT YOUR HANDS WITH LONG, THICK PLASTIC GLOVES. COVER YOUR EYES WITH GOGGLES AND DO NOT TAKE THEM OFF UNTIL YOU HAVE PUT THE SOAP IN THE MOULD. WEAR A MASK SO YOU DON'T BREATHE IN ANY FUMES.
- HAVE A PLASTIC BOTTLE WITH VINEGAR HANDY TO NEUTRALISE THE CAUSTIC SODA IN CASE OF SPILLS, AND ALSO HAVE RUNNING WATER OR A BUCKET OF WATER NEARBY (WHERE YOU WON'T TRIP OVER IT, OF COURSE).
- DO NOT HAVE LOTS OF MESS OR OBJECTS LYING AROUND THE WORKSPACE. WHEN YOU'RE FINISHED, CLEAN EVERYTHING VERY CAREFULLY.
- YOUR UTENSILS MUST BE EXCLUSIVELY USED TO MAKE SOAP..

## MATERIALS

- 2 heat-resistant plastic or glass jars (never metal)
- pot for the bain-marie
- electric stick mixer
- silicone spatula
- thermometer suitable for liquids
- goggles
- long plastic gloves
- protective mask
- precision scales
- a plastic bottle with vinegar to neutralise the soda, in the event of splashing

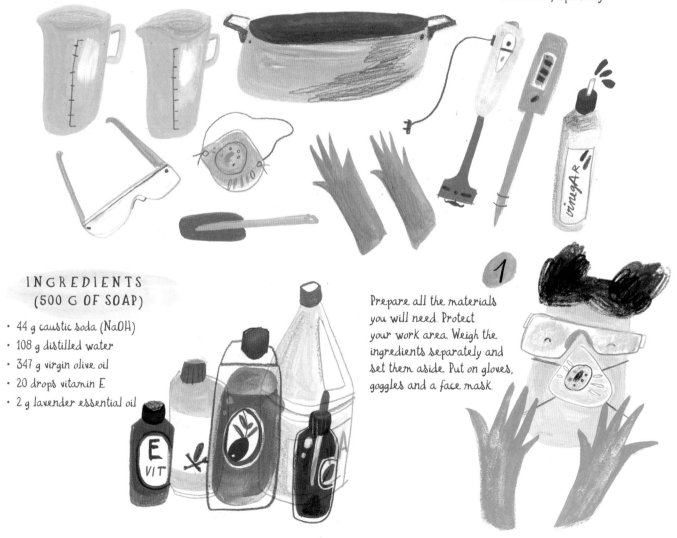

## INGREDIENTS
### (500 G OF SOAP)

- 44 g caustic soda (NaOH)
- 108 g distilled water
- 347 g virgin olive oil
- 20 drops vitamin E
- 2 g lavender essential oil

**1**

Prepare all the materials you will need. Protect your work area. Weigh the ingredients separately and set them aside. Put on gloves, goggles and a face mask.

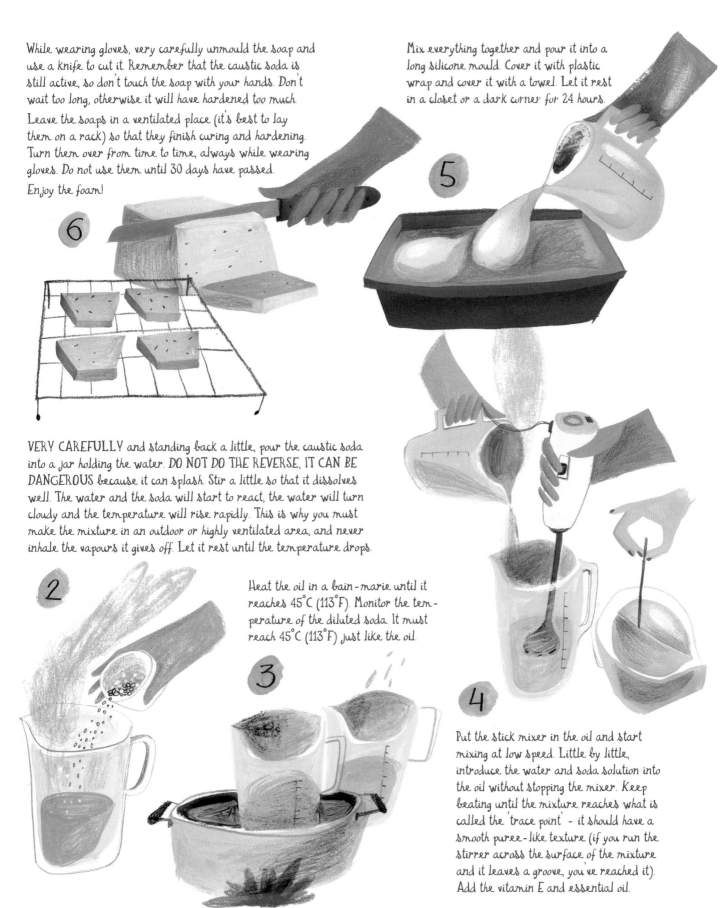

While wearing gloves, very carefully unmould the soap and use a knife to cut it. Remember that the caustic soda is still active, so don't touch the soap with your hands. Don't wait too long, otherwise it will have hardened too much.

Leave the soaps in a ventilated place (it's best to lay them on a rack) so that they finish curing and hardening. Turn them over from time to time, always while wearing gloves. Do not use them until 30 days have passed.

Enjoy the foam!

6

Mix everything together and pour it into a long silicone mould. Cover it with plastic wrap and cover it with a towel. Let it rest in a closet or a dark corner for 24 hours.

5

VERY CAREFULLY and standing back a little, pour the caustic soda into a jar holding the water. DO NOT DO THE REVERSE, IT CAN BE DANGEROUS because it can splash. Stir a little so that it dissolves well. The water and the soda will start to react, the water will turn cloudy and the temperature will rise rapidly. This is why you must make the mixture in an outdoor or highly ventilated area, and never inhale the vapours it gives off. Let it rest until the temperature drops.

2

Heat the oil in a bain-marie until it reaches 45°C (113°F). Monitor the temperature of the diluted soda. It must reach 45°C (113°F) just like the oil.

3

4

Put the stick mixer in the oil and start mixing at low speed. Little by little, introduce the water and soda solution into the oil without stopping the mixer. Keep beating until the mixture reaches what is called the 'trace point' - it should have a smooth puree-like texture (if you run the stirrer across the surface of the mixture and it leaves a groove, you've reached it). Add the vitamin E and essential oil.

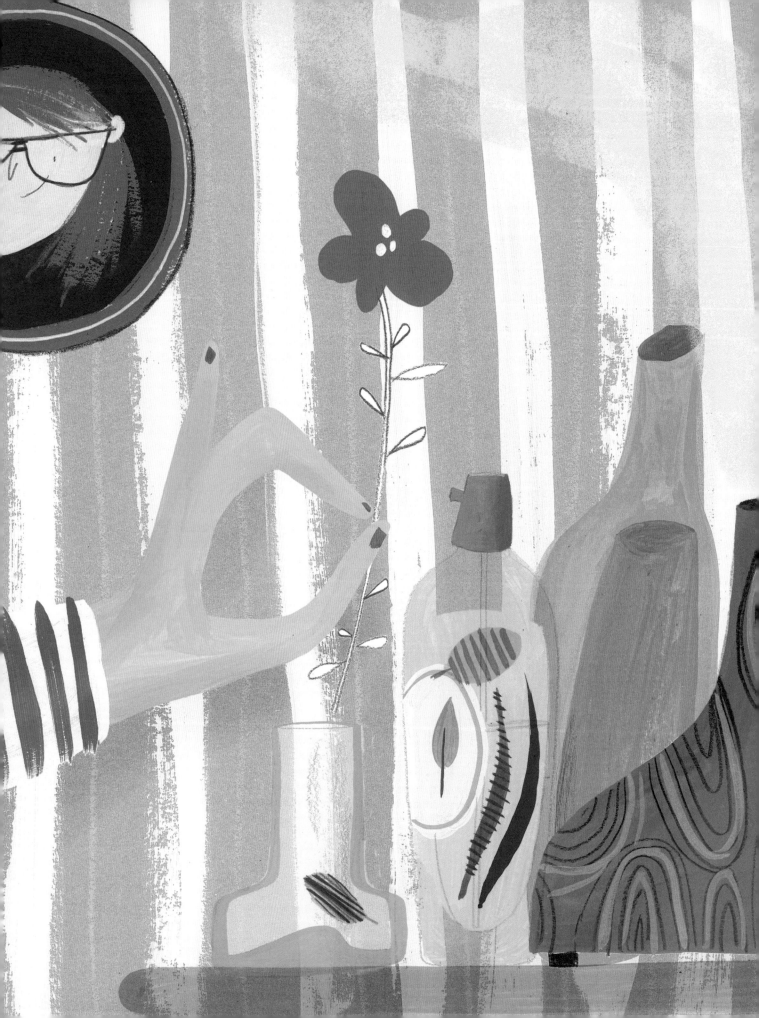

# Extras

We can use organic ingredients not only to take care of our skin and hair, but also to take care of our environment. In this chapter, I've included some extra recipes for cleaning and caring for the spaces and objects in your home.

We should reflect on whether we need so many different cleaning products for specific things. The market is crammed with detergents, softeners, corrosive agents, aerosols, air fresheners ... It doesn't take much to replace them with more environmentally friendly products. Industrial vinegar, baking soda, borax, citric acid and mild soap solutions in very hot water are more than enough to clean most of the spaces in our homes, and we can use essential oils to disinfect and create a relaxing environment.

Now that we are almost at the end, I want to preface this last chapter by thanking you for having come this far. I hope you have enjoyed this book that I have prepared with so much love. I've had a lot of fun doing it and I've learned millions of things.

I hope you liked it and that, at least, it has piqued your curiosity about making your own cosmetics.

And remember, being well inside comes first.

Thank you, thank you, thank you!

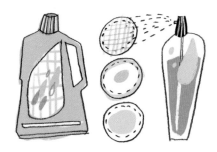

## YOGA MAT SPRAY
## OM SHANTI/NAMASTE

This spray will keep your yoga mat clean of bacteria and its aromatherapy effects will help you in your daily life. You can make different scents depending on whether you want a relaxing or energising fragrance. Mix ingredients in a spray bottle. Shake well before use. You can also use it to disinfect the inside of your sports shoes, the inside of your suitcases, cabinets, etc.

### INGREDIENTS

- distilled water
- witch-hazel hydrosol
- 1 teaspoon baking soda
- 10 g vodka (optional)

Essential oils for om shanti (relaxing) spray
- lavender
- frankincense

Essential oils for namaste (energising) spray
- tea tree
- grapefruit or tangerine

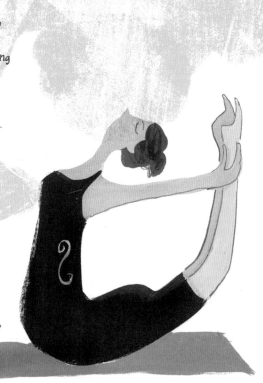
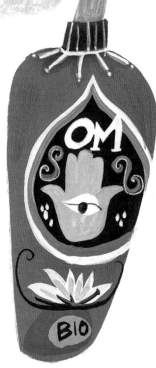
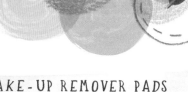

## MAKE-UP REMOVER PADS

A practical way to remove make-up wherever you are. Make a mixture with the following ingredients:

- 200 g hydrosol (lavender, rose or witch-hazel)
- 15 g liquid Castile soap
- 5 g vegetable glycerine
- 30 g vegetable oil (almond or olive)

Put the hydrosol, soap and glycerine in a container then add the oil. Mix it all very well. Place as many make-up remover pads as you can into a glass jar (without filling it too tightly) and add the make-up remover mixture so that the discs absorb it. Use a recycled plastic container to carry them when you travel.

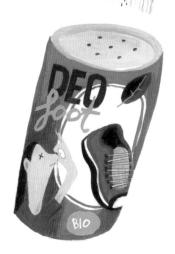

## DEODORANT POWDER
## FOR SHOES

These powders will disinfect your shoes and trainers, and help remove moisture and odours. Mix the ingredients well and transfer them to an empty talcum powder bottle or a clean spice shaker. Sprinkle inside shoes when required.

### INGREDIENTS

- 35 g fine powdered kaolin (white clay)
- 45 g cornflour (cornstarch) or arrowroot
- 10 g baking soda
- 10 drops lemon essential oil
- 5 drops mint essential oil
- 5 drops tea tree essential oil

## TANGERINE DREAM PILLOW MIST

Pillow mists or sprays set the mood and relax you due to the presence of essential oils. Spray a few times around your pillow before going to bed. If you do not have an essential oil solubiliser, you must shake the mixture very well before using it.

### INGREDIENTS

- 30 g distilled water
- 30 g vodka
- 30 g lavender or chamomile hydrosol
- 10 drops lavender essential oil
- 5 drops tangerine essential oil
- 5 drops chamomile essential oil
- approximately 10 g solubiliser

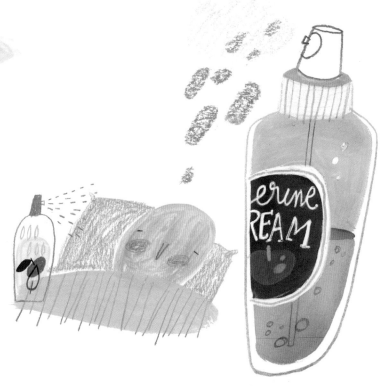

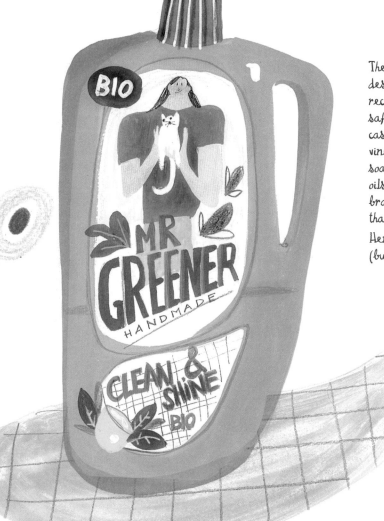

## MISTER GREENER MULTIPURPOSE CLEANER

The subject of chemicals in household cleaning products deserves an entire book. There are hundreds of recipes and alternatives to keep your house clean and safe rather than using toxic products that, in most cases, are not necessary. Lemon juice, baking soda, vinegar, citric acid, hydrogen peroxide, borax, Castile soap, even very hot water combined with essential oils, are powerful cleaners. There are also many brands that manufacture household cleaning products that respect the environment and your health.

Here's a recipe for a basic all-purpose cleaner (but for marble, use vinegar). In a spray bottle mix:

### INGREDIENTS

- 50 g white vinegar
- 15 g baking soda
- 15 g cleaning alcohol (or vinegar)
- 15 drops lemon essential oil
- 5 drops tea tree essential oil

If you want to smooth it out, add a bit of distilled water. Shake well before use.

This book is dedicated to all the women who struggle
to feel free and happy with their bodies and their lives.

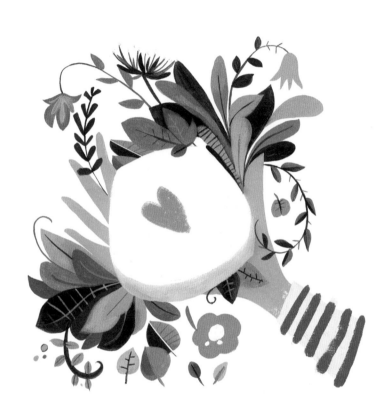

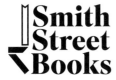

Original title: *Belleza orgánica.*
First published in 2019 by Editorial GG, SL, Barcelona, Spain
© Maru Godas /Editorial GG, SL, 2019

This edition published in 2023 by Smith Street Books
Naarm (Melbourne) | Australia
smithstreetbooks.com

ISBN: 978-1-9227-5478-3

Smith Street Books respectfully acknowledges the Wurundjeri People of the Kulin Nation,
who are the Traditional Owners of the land on which we work, and we pay our respects to
their Elders past and present.

The information in this book has been complied by way of general guidance in relation to
the specific subjects addressed, but it is not a substitute and not intended to be relied upon
for medical, healthcare or other professional advice on specific circumstances. The authors
and the publishers disclaim, as far as the law allows, any liability arising directly or indirectly
from the use or misuse of the information and recipes contained in this book.

Layout and cover art: Maru Godas

For Smith Street Books
Publisher: Paul McNally
Editor: Lorna Hendry
Proofreader: Pamela Dunne
Translation: Aisling Coughlan

Printed & bound in China by C&C Offset Printing Co., Ltd.

Book 277
10 9 8 7 6 5 4 3 2 1

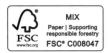

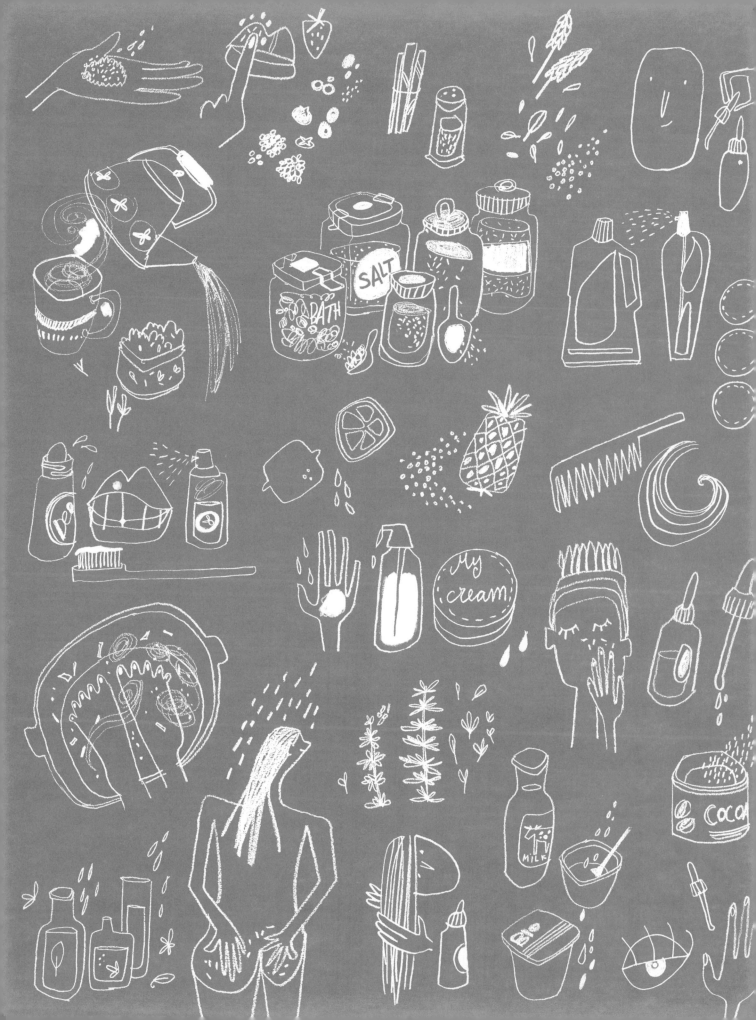